CBD Oil for Pain Relief

A Comprehensive Beginner's Guide to Learn and Understand CBD oil for pain relief

I0425536

Author: Herman Kynaston

Table of Contents

Book Description:

Are you ready to learn the truth about the healing properties of CBD oil? Pain, trauma and anxiety are greatly improved with ongoing cannabidiol treatment – and now science tells us why.

CBD oil was once banned and seen as an illegal substance across the world. Today, science has revealed the outstanding healing properties of the cannabis plant, and the non-psychoactive oils that are created from it. Finally, an effective, low impact way to treat major illnesses!

In *CBD Oil for Pain Relief,* I give you a much-needed primer on the use of CBD oil in medicine. Once you're up to speed, I review how the oil can be used to effectively treat a wide variety of chronic illnesses. This is the guide you need if you're considering CBD Oil to treat your pain.

In this book you'll learn:

- How to effectively use CBD oil for its many health benefits

- How CBD oil is extracted and the different methods used

- The types of CBD oil and how to test for quality

- If CBD really works for pain relief and exactly how

- How to treat a wide variety of ailments and disease with CBD oil

- About the precautions and side effects involved

- Good to know CBD oil recipes that are also delicious

This beginner's guide will teach you everything you need to know, if you plan on using CBD oil to treat your pain. Join people all over the world who are living with less pain thanks to CBD oil!

Learn the ins and outs of using this incredible medicine and start your own healing journey. This is the information you've been searching for.

Discover the power of CBD oil in this guide.

Get the book and start your recovery!

Introduction

"Make the most you can of the Indian Hemp seed and sow it everywhere."

- George Washington

CBD or "cannabidiol" was discovered around the 1940s. Dr. Roger Adams discovered CBD at the University of Illinois – more than twenty years before THC (the other major constituent in marijuana) was discovered. The entire structure of CBD was not elucidated until 1963. Cannabis itself has been used medicinally since as early as 1400-2000 BC.

William Osler is said to have created the first program for the medicinal use of cannabis. In 1937, cannabis was on its way to being used for industrial and medicinal purposes with the "Marijuana Tax Act." Cannabis was then criminalized in 1969, and the act was ruled unconstitutional. For quite some time, the research in the United States regarding the medicinal benefits of cannabis stopped.

In 1998, a company called GW Pharmaceuticals, based in Cambridge, United Kingdom began growing cannabis in order to use it for clinical trials. The goal was to produce CBD-rich plants and in turn, produce a medicine that had little to no psychoactive effects. A "CBD-rich" plant is considered to have at least 4 percent CBD (dry weight). The CBD-rich plants not only countered the psychoactive effects of THC but also had their own benefits.

GW Pharmaceuticals was given access to HortaPharm, a Dutch seed company's genetic library.

CBD is a naturally occurring cannabinoid. In hemp plants there are at least 130 cannabinoids - CBD is one of them and takes up to 40 percent of the plant's extract. When it was first discovered, it was not thought to be pharmaceutically active.

CBD oil is taken from the flowers, stems, leaves or buds (resin glands) of marijuana (cannabis) or taken from hemp. It is commonly thought that CBD taken from marijuana is of better quality and concentration because it contains complementary cannabinoids. The flowers are going to be the most valuable due to their density, creating a full spectrum oil. Full spectrum CBD oil of high quality is often made with only the female flowers.

Hemp is a fibrous, industrial form of cannabis. Hemp has little tiny buds and a THC (tetrahydrocannabinol) level of 0.3 percent or less. CBD oil usually contains another type of oil such as MCT oil. THC is what gets you high or produces the euphoric and intoxicating feelings. CBD oil will not get you "high," because it contains little to no THC.

Oddly enough, our bodies actually make their own cannabinoids and have a system to make them work together properly. For example, you should think of cannabinoids as little soldiers fighting along in your body. It is their job to make sure everything is balanced inside. Every living thing with a vertebrate has an endocannabinoid system (ECS). It is the endocannabinoid system that makes the cannabinoids or "soldiers."

The endocannabinoid system is still something many are unaware of. It is newly discovered within the animal and human body. The endocannabinoid system has very specific duties, much like our nervous system and immune system. The endocannabinoid system, as stated, is in charge of maintaining balance in the body, along with regulating homeostasis. It does things like regulating our mood, memory, pain perception, sleep, motor control, appetite, and more. The endocannabinoid system does so by producing the cannabinoids or "soldiers."

As we grow older, our endocannabinoid system begins to wear out – much like everything else within our bodies. As this happens, the endocannabinoid system starts to have trouble maintaining balance. Fewer cannabinoids are made, and you can even become cannabinoid deficient. The endocannabinoid system can also be disrupted if a person is sick, has a disease or is injured.

Unfortunately, once the body begins to run low on cannabinoids, there is not typically a "natural" way to get more. In fact, the last time you got cannabinoids was from your mother's milk during infancy (that is if you were breastfed). You probably are not going to have access to "mother's milk" at this stage in your life, so what gives? This is where the cannabis/hemp plant comes into play.

Plant-based cannabinoids stimulate your endocannabinoid system naturally by reinforcing it. In other terms, these cannabinoids or "plant soldiers" stimulate the body's natural defenses, which soothe your ailment. This allows the body to rebalance. Having an out of balance body can surface in many forms such as having chronic anxiety.

The best part of plant-based cannabinoids is that they are completely natural, given to us from the earth. They are not man-made, artificial, mixed with chemicals or physically addictive.

CBD works by exerting itself through several pathways. One site is the system of receptors found in the central and peripheral nervous systems, brain, muscle, fat and immune cells, called the endocannabinoid system. Although THC activates the endocannabinoid system stronger, the way CBD acts is more complex. Both constituents bind themselves to CB in the endocannabinoid receptor. CBD likely inhibits the release of glutamate, which is an excitatory neurotransmitter. The CB receptor is in charge of maintaining normal brain activity, such as protecting against seizures.

It is the CBD's interactions in the endocannabinoid system that counteracts the effects of THC, which are physiological and psychological. CBD also increases anandamide, an endocannabinoid. Anandamide has anti-inflammatory effects. Additionally, there is a biochemical target of CBD that is the TRP (transient receptor potential) class of channels. This affects calcium levels in the cell and can increase calcium levels in other cells as well.

The signaling of the 5HT-1A serotonin receptor is increased by CBD. Serotonin is found in the body, and it regulates the mood. What the CBD does is decrease anxiety. It protects the brain from oxidative stress, inflammation and increases levels of adenosine. Adenosine is a neurotransmitter and molecule that helps with sleep regulation and energy creation. A serotonin dysfunction is often due to depression or a number of other disorders.

In simpler terms, CBD helps the body with emotional and physical stress due to changes in the immediate environment by maintaining homeostasis.

There is a whole-plant CBD-rich oil and a single-molecule CBD. Single-molecule CBD is going to be less therapeutically effective. It lacks important secondary cannabinoids and other medicinal compounds.

CBD products typically fall into three categories. Crystalline isolate, which contains zero THC; unrefined full spectrum, which contains some THC but less than 0.3 percent, along with CBN and CBG; and full spectrum, which contains some THC but less than 0.3 percent.

Crystalline isolate has the appearance of salt crystals. The benefit is they have no taste and they do not contain any THC. The negative side of crystalline isolate is that it has no plant nutrients, making it a weak product. Essentially you need to consume a lot of the product to feel its CBD effects.

Unrefined full spectrum is very thick, cloudy and dark. The THC in unrefined full spectrum products amplifies the CBD effects. Unrefined full spectrum also has many other plant nutrients and cannabinoids such as CBN, CBG, CBDV, terpenes, omega 3, omega 6, omega 9 and plant sterols. Unrefined full spectrum can be called "rick system style," meaning it is dark, raw and full of nutrients. However, with unrefined full spectrum, there is a certain amount of THC present. Unrefined full spectrum can also have an earthy, unpleasant taste. It is important to get an unrefined full-spectrum product that has been properly flavored by the company who makes it.

Full spectrum oil is gold or see-through, to clear. The benefit of full spectrum products is that it is less refined than crystalline iodine, but has some THC as well. The THC helps with the CBD effects, making the product more effective. This is sometimes called the "entourage effect." Full spectrum products can taste unpleasant, so again it is important to get a full spectrum product that has been properly flavored.

CBD oil has continued to gain popularity since the legalization of recreational marijuana in Colorado and Washington in 2012. Since then, several other states have also legalized recreational marijuana use, only adding to the popularity of CBD oil.

In the past several years, CBD has continued to gain momentum in the health and wellness community. This is in part due to scientific studies proving the amazing benefits and potential that CBD contains.

Chapter 1
Health Benefits of CBD Oil

"We shall, by and by, want a world of hemp more for our own consumption."

- John Adams

CBD is just one of 100+ cannabinoids in cannabis. It has numerous health benefits including pain relief, help with epilepsy and help with sleeping problems. CBD oil can be used in treating cancer patients and much, much more.

Additionally, CBD is non-psychoactive, so you are not going to get "high" when consuming it. This makes it safer and more appealing to those worried about the mind-altering effects that THC can have.

Pain relief is one of the most highly regarded health benefits of CBD oil due to its analgesic effects. Apparently, CBD interacts with brain receptors and the immune system; this alleviates pain and reduces inflammation. Several studies have been conducted proving that CBD reduces inflammation within mice and rats.

Chronic inflammation is a large problem in our society that leads to many non-infectious diseases including cancer, Alzheimer's, heart disease, and autoimmune diseases, to name a few. A healthy diet and lifestyle are going to do wonders with chronic inflammation, but when a person is already doing both, along with getting good sleep and exercise, CBD oil can be an added bonus on top. Research has proven that CBD oil has the ability to reduce chronic inflammation that can lead to a disease.

More technically, CBD has the ability to blunt Th1 and Th2 dominance

In a study with rats with asthma, Th1 (TNF-a and IL-6) and Th2 (IL-4, IL-5, Il-13) responses were reduced after being treated with CBD.

CBD decreased the release and production of inflammatory cytokines like Th1 (IFN-gamma, TNF-alpha, and IL-6), Th2 (IL-4) and IL-8.

CBD has the ability to suppress Th17 dominance, meaning it can help with Th-17-dominant autoimmune diseases.

More anti-inflammatory mechanisms CBD has includes reducing the mobilization and growth of neutrophils and reducing the inflammatory Macrophage Inflammatory Protein-1 (MIP-1 beta, MIP-1 alpha)

Studies show that CBD is an effective pain-relief treatment that causes no negative side effects in patients. Those who particularly suffer from fibromyalgia and multiple sclerosis can find pain relief in CBD oil. It is recommended for those with multiple sclerosis, to take a combination of CBD and THC. It will effectively treat muscle tightness, sleep disturbances, loss of bladder control (urinary incontinence), and pain.

CBD oil can be particularly helpful to those with rheumatoid arthritis; this is due to its anti-inflammatory effects. The CBD can help with swelling, joint pain, disease progression, and decrease joint destruction – this can lead to better quality of sleep. No negative side effects were discovered.

CBD oil can even prevent nervous system degeneration. The best part of CBD oil is that it does not allow one to develop a tolerance or become dependent on it like many opioids do. CBD oil is a wonderful choice for those who are looking to stay away from highly addictive opioids.

Epilepsy is another major thing that CBD oil can help with. Epilepsy causes excessive and abnormal brain cell activity; due to this, disturbance seizures occur. There have been many major newsworthy cases over the years that have brought attention to CBD oil for its anti-seizure properties.

More recently there have been studies done to back up these cases, showing that CBD oil is actually effective with epilepsy. Specifically, there is one form of epilepsy, Dravet Syndrome, which can be treated effectively with CBD oil. Dravet Syndrome is an uncommon form of epilepsy that is often induced by fever. Those with Dravet Syndrome who participated in the study conducted by The New England Journal of Medicine, and experienced reduced seizures. In this placebo-controlled, randomized, double-blind study, a median seizure frequency dropped by 38.9 percent.

In another survey that included children and their parents, 84 percent of the parents reported back that their children's seizure frequency reduced by 84 percent. These kids also experienced elevated mood, better sleep, and increased alertness. The only side effects were fatigue and drowsiness.

In addition, after three months of treatment with CBD oil, 39 percent of the kids had more than 50 percent reduction in their seizures.

CBD oil is also effective in treating some mental health conditions, most commonly anxiety. One study showed that, in particular, CBD oil can help with social anxiety disorder, post-traumatic stress disorder (PTSD) and obsessive-compulsive disorder. It also helps with the fear of public speaking.

Depression is another mental health condition that CBD oil can help with. It has been shown to do so by enhancing glutamate cortical signaling and serotonergic cortical signaling. Those with depression have a lack of both of those forms of cortical signaling.

CBD and schizophrenia

Schizophrenia is a complex and serious disease. This disease is most commonly managed with prescription medications and therapy. Unfortunately, many of the medications have negative side effects. CBD oil has been shown to lessen hallucinations in those with schizophrenia.

A March 2015 review stated that CBD oil is a harmless, effective and well-tolerated treatment for psychosis. However, more research needs to be done. Although CBD oil should be safe, THC may not be safe for those with schizophrenia.

CBD oil can help fight cancer! Studies have recently shown that CBD oil can be highly valuable in treating cancer. CBD and other compounds in cannabis can kill tumor cells in colon cancer and leukemia. The CBD reduces human glioma cell invasion and growth, proving it can be an anti-tumor agent. CBD oil has also shown to stop the spreading of cancer cells in cervical cancer.

It is thought that CBD can also be used as a tool in combination therapy for prostate cancer and breast cancer (again, this is due to the CBD's anti-tumor effects). The CBD can also improve the effectiveness of the typical anti-tumor drugs that are being used, and also help with pain reduction.

- CBD can decrease the ability of cancer cells to produce energy – this leads to their death

- CBD treatment helps the LAK (lymphokine-activated killer) cells to kill cancer cells more effectively

- CBD blocks CPR55 signaling which decreases cancer cell proliferation

However, most studies done on CBD oil and cancer are still under what is called "pre-clinical," which means they were not conducted on humans or mammals. It is just important to be mindful of CBD oil having the 100 percent ability to cure cancer.

CBD oil can help stimulate genes and proteins that help break down fat, maintain healthy blood sugar, and increase mitochondria that will help burn calories. Additionally, CBD oil will encourage the body to change white fat to brown fat. White fat is the most common kind of body fat and is the classical form of "fat" we think of. Brown fat is a small fat deposit, and it acts differently than white fat. Brown fat is not considered bad; in fact, it is said to improve health. It improves the body's ability to burn the white fat, regulates blood sugar and creates heat.

Less commonly, CBD oil can reduce the risk of diabetes. A Neuropharmacology study showed that only 32 percent of a group of non-obese, diabetes-prone mice who were given CBD, developed diabetes. In the group of non-obese, diabetes-prone mice that were not given CBD 100 percent of them developed diabetes.

Another less common benefit of CBD oil is its ability to fight multi-drug resistant bacteria. A study done in 2011 showed that CBD oil helped slow the progression of tuberculosis in rats. CBD does not possess antibacterial properties; it inhibits T-cell proliferation. This is important as more and more "superbugs" come about that are antibiotic-resistant, we are running out of options. CBD may be one, powerful option.

In the United States, heart disease is the primary cause of death, and CBD oil can help that. Obviously, leading a healthy lifestyle and eating a healthy diet are most important in combating heart disease, but CBD oil can also be effective. Research has been done that shows that cannabidiol can reduce artery blockage, blood pressure, cholesterol and stress-induced cardiovascular response.

CBD oil can be used as a treatment with Crohn's disease – something that affects 200,000 Americans each year, while in North America, more than half a million people. Crohn's disease is an inflammatory bowel disorder. It causes sores and ulcers in the digestive tract. Symptoms include diarrhea, weight loss, abdominal pain, bloody stools and sometimes skin and eye conditions. It is most common in men ages 15 to 30 and has no cure. Crohn's disease can be treated by managing symptoms with medications, but it is not always so easy. Many of the medications have severely negative side effects that can sometimes be worse than the symptoms that come with having Crohn's disease. The cons associated with traditional Crohn's disease medications include a high rate of addiction (typically associated with opioids).

CBD has the ability to reduce inflammatory hypermotility, which is associated with diseases such as Crohn's. CBD inhibits a liver enzyme that breaks down endocannabinoids, allowing anandamide to exert its natural anti-inflammatory and anti-motility effects.

This is beneficial to those with Crohn's disease, due to how common gastrointestinal infections are.

CBD oil can help your skin! Topical CBD creams can treat many skin conditions like eczema, by encouraging abnormal cell death. CBD can also help with acne by decreasing lipid synthesis and proliferation of human sebaceous glands. CBD also has an anti-inflammatory effect on sebaceous glands, so it has the potential to treat acne vulgaris. CBD oil also reduces the growth of keratinocytes (skin cells); this can help with psoriasis. CBD oil can help regulate the skin's oil production. Vitamin E has always been known to be great for the skin, and CBD oil contains it!

CBD oil can increase appetite, along with relieving vomiting and nausea. This was shown in a study with rats. However, it can be complex, because the CBD helped with vomiting and nausea when the rats were given toxic drugs. When the rats were given high doses of CBD, nausea increased or had no effect.

CBD can bind to cannabinoid receptors in the body, which increase appetite, according to the National Cancer Institute. And for those with food sensitivities, CBD oil helped eliminate them – a small but wonderful improvement in everyday life.

CBD oil has the potential to help one quit smoking, and help with drug withdrawals. A study done by Addictive Behaviors, an international peer journal, showed that smokers who used a CBD inhaler smoked fewer cigarettes throughout the day. The inhaler contained the CBD compound helped curb cravings for nicotine.

Other studies done in the United Kingdom by the University College in London had similar results. In this 2013 study, dependent smokers were given a CBD inhaler to use upon having a nicotine craving. It was shown that their cigarette intake reduced by 40 percent. Those dependent smokers who were given a placebo inhaler did not have a significant reduction in their cigarette intake.

A more recent study done in the United Kingdom in May 2018, also showed that those given an 800mg dose of CBD had significant reductions in cigarette cravings.

Cigarette smoking goes beyond being a physical addiction; it is also a habit that has to be broken. Smoking CBD oil could be a similar substitute that relieves anxiety.

Using CBD oil as a substitute in place of smoking cigarettes is a great alternative because it is a non-intoxicating compound that does not get you high and has a lot of medical benefits.

A study done by Neurotherapeutics showed that CBD can be a good substance for those abusing opioids. CBD has the capabilities to be a good "exit drug." An exit drug has the ability to wean someone off opioids. CBD can do so by helping with the pain that usually, initially, got them addicted to opioids in the first place and by helping with opioid withdrawal symptoms.

A June 2017 study titled, Cannabis As A Substitute For Opioid-Based Pain Medication: Patient Self-Report, where data was collected from nearly 3000 medical cannabis patient, showed that people with access to CBD took fewer prescription opioids for pain. It is also true that doctors prescribe fewer opiates for the pain to people in states that have accessible medical CBD. More obviously, these states also have fewer opioid hospitalizations and fewer overdose deaths.

CBD can help many kinds of recovering addicts. Studies have shown the same, with other substances such as cocaine and alcohol.

A recent Nature study done in March 2018 showed that CBD oil could be successful in treating addiction in animals. Alcohol or cocaine-addicted rats were given CBD oil topically once a day for a week. The research showed that these rats were less likely to relapse, even while in stressful situations. The study also showed that the rats had reduced impulsivity and anxiety, two traits commonly associated with addiction.

The study went on, to show that the CBD oil had worked on the rats even five months later, even though it was out of their systems. The rats were still less likely to relapse in stressful situations or when provoked by "drug cues" because they had been treated with CBD oil.

CBD oil can even work effectively with animals. Mammals have an endocannabinoid system, just like us humans; therefore, CBD oil can give them the same benefits it gives us.

In cats and dogs CBD oil can help with pain, increasing appetite, getting along with other pets, separation anxiety, excessive crying or barking, and relaxation (maybe for a vet trip).

To successfully give your pet CBD oil, you need to find the right dosage for them (just as you'd do with yourself). Start out with a small dosage. A good rule of thumb is 1 milligram for every 10 pounds of their body weight. Eventually, you can level up to 5 milligrams per 10 pounds of body weight. Sometimes you will even have to give a bit more for a more serious condition, such as an excessive pain that your pet is going through. It is recommended to give your pet their CBD oil spread-out, throughout the day – 3-4 times. This is more effective than just giving them one large dose each day.

CBD Oil Benefits Technically Explained

- CBD will activate 5HT1A receptors and 5HT2A receptors (slightly)

- Activating 5HT1A receptors helps with vomiting and nausea, depression, appetite, anxiety, addictions, and sleep

- CBD takes part in the perception of inflammation and pain by activating the TRPV-1 receptor

- CBD is capable of blocking FAAH enzyme and anandamide reuptake, which indirectly activates CB1 receptors and increases the level of anandamide, making it effective against depression and anxiety

- CBD can reduce seizures by modulating neuron excitability and intracellular Ca2+ ions

The most common of those is ingestion (taking it orally) – you can do this with a concentrated paste or a tincture/drop format. It is important to first hold it under the tongue, so it is absorbed in the mouth. The digestive system breaks some of the CBD down.

The objective is simply that the cannabinoids enter your system easily to achieve the results you want. How you take the CBD oil usually relates to how much you are taking, or the "dosage," and how long you want the effects to last.

It seems most people that take CBD oil do not prefer the method most similar to smoking, which is vaping. However, when taking CBD oil by vaping the effects occur quite quicker – within a few minutes, compared to what can be hours.

Additionally, when taking CBD oil in a manner that does not allow the effects to occur until later, the effects often last longer.

If you decide to take CBD oil orally, you will do so by taking capsules, edibles or adding it to the food or drinks you are already consuming. You can also take CBD oil in the form of tincture. You take tincture by placing small drops of it in your mouth, directly under your tongue or adding it to your food or drink. A lot of people prefer a tincture, because of how discreet it is.

CBD oil tinctures sometimes referred to as "drops" come as liquid supplements. They are packaged in a glass bottle with a dropper or spray top to make for easily dispensing. As stated before, the tincture form is very popular. An added factor to that is the ingredients that can be added. Manufacturers often add coconut oil, spearmint, terpenes, essential oils or natural herbs. These all do wonders in masking the potent taste of CBD oil.

When taking CBD oil tincture, use your dropper top to suck up as much CBD oil as desired, and then place it under your tongue. Wait about a minute to a minute and a half to swallow the CBD oil tincture. If the flavor is too much for you, you can try drinking some juice alongside swallowing the CBD oil tincture.

There are many, many types of CBD oil tinctures – varying in flavor, strength, and size. If you do not like one specific kind, think about trying something else before throwing in the towel with tinctures.

Some CBD oil is made for vaping pens, which is going to be the method that allows you to feel the effects of the CBD the quickest. When you vape CBD oil, it enters your bloodstream directly through your lungs.

When vaping CBD oil or e-liquid, you will need a vaporizer or vape pen. Buying a vape kit is also an option. A vape kit includes a disposable vape cartridge that will screw into the vaporizer. With a disposable vaporizer pen, you do not have to worry about the hassle of maintaining your vaporizer pen. A regular vaporizer pen will need its tank and coils replaced once in a while. There are many vaping products out there – many of them affordable and disposable!

Vaping CBD oil should not be as harmful as smoking cigarettes. Vaping CBD oil can actually be seen as a sort of relaxing. One CBD oil consumer who vapes said, "When I'm feeling anxious, or in serious need of relaxation, I immediately grab my vaporizer." When you vape, you are inhaling and exhaling. Its two practices many people use to achieve peace and calmness, a bit like performing a type of calming, breathing technique that one may do while meditating or practicing yoga.

Sublingual sprays are also discreet like the tincture form.

Topical CBD creams are most effective for those with joint or muscle pain. Topical CBD creams are also popular with those who have inflamed, dry or aging skin. Our skin is actually our largest organ, so topical CBD creams are a great way to take care of it through balance and moisturization properly.

Obviously, topical CBD creams are only to be used externally. You will want to apply them to the target areas – such as where you are in pain, or where your dry skin is located. Using topical CBD creams is super simple. You simply massage the targeted area with the product, much like applying lotion or sunscreen.

Topical CBD creams have anti-inflammatory and pain relieving properties. They can help those who have arthritis. There are many topical CBD products out there that vary in consistency.

Another form, in which CBD oil is often consumed, is a pure concentrate. It is a paste-like oil, extracted from the hemp plant. Most likely, your pure concentrate CBD oil will be packaged in an oral syringe, which can be a bit intimidating for some, or may simply be unappealing, but never fear. You do not actually inject the CBD oil.

Squeeze out from the syringe as much CBD oil as you plan to take onto either the back of a spoon, directly under your tongue, or finger. The end result will be placing the CBD oil under your tongue – it is up to you how it gets there!

The reason the CBD oil is placed under the tongue is that, in the mouth, there are capillary glands that absorb the oil. When the capillary glands absorb the CBD oil, it enters your system rapidly. When you swallow the CBD oil, a good amount of it will have already been absorbed by your body.

An average amount of CBD oil to take is about the size of a grain of rice – pretty small! You do not want to over-do it. Better to be safe than sorry. So try not to get too much. If anything squeezes less than needed and then you can always squeeze out more.

It is important to be careful during this step because CBD oil when in a pure concentrated form, is a natural oil. Each one is going to vary in its consistency and its flavor. Sometimes the pure concentrate is runny; sometimes it is very thick. If you get something totally dissimilar to what you had before, that is perfectly normal. However, the CBD oil pure concentrate can stain, so be careful when getting it out of the syringe. You do not want to get any on your clothes, floors, or surfaces in your home.

Once the CBD oil pure concentrate is under your tongue, you want to wait a minute or a minute and a half to swallow it. The longer you wait, typically the better the results, this is recommended by most but it really is your call and what you feel most comfortable with.

Be warned that CBD oil does not taste "good." One CBD oil consumer said "pure hemp oil tastes like you grabbed a handful of dirt and grass and ate it. Sometimes it is a little spicy, too." If you simply cannot get over the taste, it is recommended that you take CBD oil sublingually, but it is believed that CBD oil taken in a pure concentrate form is the best way to get a large number of cannabinoids in your system, each day.

One way to get around the "bad" taste of CBD oil in pure concentrate form is to try drinking juice as you swallow it. Apple cider and orange juice seem to be most effective at masking the potent taste of the CBD oil pure concentrate.

As stated before, the CBD oil is going to vary in its consistency and taste due to the harvest. With each harvest will bring a different taste due to terpenes - compounds in the hemp plant. Much like cannabinoids, it is not possible to tell what compounds have formed in the plant until the oil has actually been extracted and then tested. There really is no way to say how a batch will taste until it is already made.

It is hard to know how much CBD oil to take, especially when it is your first time using it. Unfortunately, there is so no standard dosage, and we are all different. The proper dosage for you may not be the proper dosage for everyone else. Our bodies are all very unique, so you are the only one who can adjust your own dosage.

The FDA allows CBD oil to be sold by manufacturers as a food supplement, not as a type of medicinal product. It will not be until CBD oil is sold as a remedy or medicinal supplement, that we will ever have any scientific data that supports specific dosages.

Since the FDA has to treat CBD oil as a food supplement, it has a type of nutritional label, similar to the ones you see on food items. A requirement of food labels is having a "suggested serving size." Unfortunately, this is a bit of a disservice to consumers of CBD oil since our bodies are all vastly different. The suggested serving size number is arbitrary and should not be regarded, in most cases.

For example, when starting out with CBD oil, it is recommended to start with a smaller dosage. It is important to not take a dosage amount you saw online. Use information online as a guide and not as a personalized recommendation. If you are using CBD oil to treat a specific condition, and have a doctor for that condition, then they can give you professional advice regarding CBD oil usage and dosage.

It is very important to think about your current health condition – the severity, your diet and weight, metabolism and if you have a tolerance to CBD already. For example, if your weight changes, your CBD dosage should also change. Metabolism does not typically change as quickly, but lifestyle changes can. If you switch up your activity levels – going from active to sedentary, you will want to think about your CBD dosage. Just remember to take all factors into account. A general rule of thumb is that the heavier you are (physically), the more CBD oil you will have to take. This also applies to the severity of the condition you are trying to treat (the more severe, the more you will have to take).

A general guide for CBD dosage depending on the severity of condition and weight is as follows:

Severity of condition 1 (mild), 2, 3 (medium), 4, 5 (severe)

Weight of person - 31 pounds – 61 pounds: 2mg – 4mg + (1, mild), 4mg – 8mg + (2), 8mg – 12mg + (3, medium), 12mg – 18mg + (4), 18mg – 30mg +(5, severe)

Weight of person - 61 pounds - 100 pounds: 4mg - 6mg + (1, mild), 6mg -12mg + (2), 12mg 18mg + (3, medium), 18mg – 24mg + (4),

24mg – 40mg + (5, severe) Weight of person - 100 pounds – 175 pounds: 6mg – 8mg + (1, mild), 8mg – 18mg + (2), 18mg – 24mg + (3, medium), 24mg – 32mg + (4), 32mg – 60mg + (5, severe)

Weight of person - 175 pounds – 250 pounds: 8mg – 10mg + (1, mild), 12mg – 20mg + (2), 22mg – 30mg + (3, medium), 32mg – 40mg + (4), 42mg – 60mg + (5, severe)

When starting out taking CBD oil, make sure to observe the effects – how you feel? It is helpful and recommended, to write down the amount of CBD oil you took, what time, your weight, what you ate that day, how you felt before taking the CBD oil, and how you felt after taking the CBD oil. You can also include anything else you find to be relevant. Make sure to do this every day.

Split up a large dose into a bunch of smaller doses, and take them throughout the day. Do this for a few days to observe the effects and see if it is working for you. You should be able to determine if you need to take less or more. Always do so gradually – take a bit more or a bit less. Large doses can often act as sedatives – making one drowsy, and small doses can act as stimulants – making one alert. You can also experience dizziness, or a dry mouth – these are the most common side effects.

Just because CBD is a natural plant extract (there are no dangerous side effects or risk of overdose), does not mean you should take as much as you like. Taking the wrong dosage will not help you with your issue(s) and can make you feel uncomfortable or bad.

On the contrary, there is no data supporting that it is possible to take "too much." A good example is eating fruits and vegetables to improve your health. It is hard to over-do it with something like that. It is not possible to overdose. You might make yourself a bit sick by overeating, but you will definitely survive. Typically, you are more in trouble when not consuming enough healthy food items (such as fruits and vegetables).

How to Use CBD

There are many different methods for consuming CBD Oil. The trick, however, is that not all methods of taking it in are the best option for everyone. This decision can be very tricky because of the many factors that can influence results. To make the right choice, all you need to do is to remember three things.

1. Taste

2. Location

3. Preference

Undoubtedly, no matter which forms you take it in, chances are you will see benefits. This is a logical result that everyone wants to receive. However, the above three factors should also have a bearing on your decision.

Some people do not realize that CBD Oil can come in a wide variety of flavors and textures, so you should have no problem finding one that suits your personal taste preferences. However, you must make sure that you're buying one that is potent enough to do the job.

Pure CBD Oil is the simplest of all the forms. It is the oil that has been extracted directly from the seeds and the stalks of the plant. When you take this pure form of CBD Oil, you have the option to ingest it, which is the fastest way of getting relief, but you will need to choose a flavor that is appealing to you so that you can maximize the results.

You can also 'vape' your oil by using an oil vape pen. This will allow you to inhale it, so it gets across the blood-brain barrier much quicker. Some even use it as a condiment or a flavoring.

Once you've determined the form and the potency you want, then by factoring in your personal preferences, you will ensure that your experience with CBD Oil will not only yield you healthy benefits but will also be a more pleasurable experience; something that is not even considered when taking traditional pharmaceuticals.

If you choose to smoke your CBD, you will get a much higher concentration of the compound. There are several ways you can smoke it:

By using an oil rig, which is used in much the same way as you would a water pipe where the oil is heated to a set temperature, filtered, and then inhaled.[1]

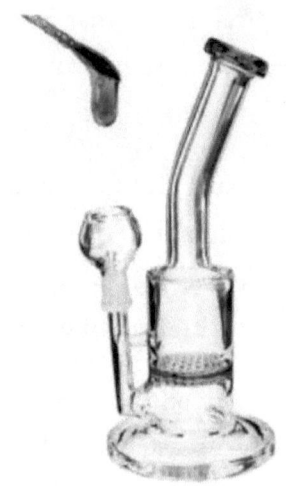

---

[1] *ALPHA BOOKS. (2019). HEAL YOURSELF WITH CBD OIL. [Place of publication not identified]: ALPHA Books.*

You can use a CBD Oil concentrate in something called dabbing. This will make it easier to harness the effects and allow you to enjoy it in a highly purified form.

When you smoke CBD Oil, it is much easier to manage your dosage, so you know exactly how much you are consuming. However, smoking also has a negative side effect of irritating your throat and lungs, which could lead to more problems later on. This could literally have a counter effect on the benefits you are trying to achieve.

Vaping CBD is one of the most popular ways of getting it into your system. Unlike smoking, it is a system that is very soothing and relaxing.

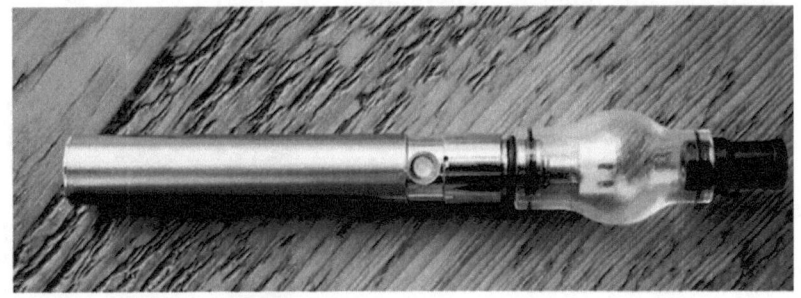

If you are not familiar with vaping, you can start with one of the more popular options, the CBD Vape-Oil, contains somewhere between 50 and 100mg of cannabidiol in each dose. Many vape starter kits can help you get the hang of it without much effort. Once you get comfortable with it, you can then move on to some of the stronger flavors that can range all the way up to 200mg (maximum dosage). Vaping provides you with a safer alternative to smoking but allows you to get the same or similar effects at the same time.

Choosing to use CBD concentrates is another option especially if you're looking for stronger results. Just keep in mind that CBD concentrates can hold as much as 10 times more cannabinoid than any other product out there, so be careful. While they are easy to calculate and measure, it is important that you know beforehand that you're getting a very powerful dosage of the substance.

Concentrates are popular among people who are busy and don't have a lot of time to wait for the weaker products to take effect.

Tinctures

If you're looking to get the product into your system very quickly, you might want to consider using a tincture. A tincture is getting the oil in an herbal liquid form that you can take orally. These tinctures are usually quite high in cannabidiol and offer quick relief.

It is important to understand though that tinctures are not pure CBD Oil, but it is oil mixed with other substances that could have a less desirable effect on your health. If you're planning to use a tincture, make sure that you know exactly what you're getting and what possible side-effects the other substances might cause. That being said, tinctures usually do have a high dosage of CBD Oil in them and can be quite strong as a result. Do not think that because it is 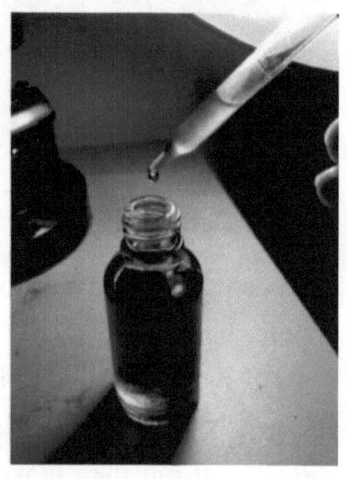 mixed with other ingredients, that you are getting a diluted form of the product. In fact, you are likely to get exactly the opposite.

Tinctures are commonly found in two different forms; a spray or a drop and their content usually range from as little as 100mg to as much as 500mg.

To take a tincture in drop form, simply place a few drops under the tongue and hold it in place for 30 seconds before swallowing. You should begin to feel an immediate soothing effect throughout the body.

One of the biggest advantages of tinctures is that you can have a powerful product that is very easy to take without any added equipment (as in vaping) that will give you near immediate results. Tinctures are also quite discreet so you wouldn't have to worry about prying eyes when taking them in public.

The additional substances used in tinctures may also leave a big question mark in your mind. Some may even contain alcohol, which comes with its own list of health concerns. If you're someone who is looking to avoid or limit your alcohol intake, it is important that you look for those tinctures containing vegetable glycerin as an alternative.

CBD Oil Topical

Topicals can be very practical when you are dealing with ailments that afflict your hair and skin. Topicals also come in many forms including salves, shampoos, and conditioners. All topicals are meant to be used externally. Even though the CBD Oil is very digestible, they could have other ingredients that may not be considered edible and could cause harm.

Salves are ideally used to treat skin conditions. They are a great way to soothe rashes, skin redness, excessive itching and similar problems that can affect your quality of life. CBD Oil found in topical treatments will help to soothe any discomfort and boost the body's natural ability to heal.

Shampoos and conditioners will treat the same conditions in the scalp area and give you healthier hair as a result, especially when used in conjunction with skin treatments. By simply applying the topical cream or salve to the affected area, you should begin to experience relief very quickly.

One of the biggest advantages to using topicals is that the skin will naturally absorb it very quickly and it can go to work on the affected area almost immediately. However, topicals are not as strong as the treatments that can be ingested or inhaled and they do not come in very high dosages so the results you receive will not only be temporary but limited.

Capsules

If you plan to take a daily supplement of CBD Oil, then the easiest way is in capsule form. It is not only precise in that you get the same dosage in each capsule, but it requires no special thought process in preparation or in measuring. This form is very practical if you lead a busy and hectic lifestyle, and is the ideal solution for those people who do not like either the taste or the smell of cannabis. Capsules are almost 100% tasteless and take only a few seconds to consume.

They can also be carried around discreetly and can be taken no matter where you are if you are traveling, so they are extremely convenient. No doubt, this is probably the most preferred method of CBD Oil compared to any others. The only drawback is that they may not be the best option for anyone who has trouble swallowing pills as they could be very difficult to get down.

Edible Form

You've probably already heard of cookies, brownies and other food products that have been made with CBD Oil. These are likely a favorite of those who don't mind spending a little more time in the kitchen to make taking their dosage more pleasant.

Unlike any other form of medical treatment, to get CBD Oil in the right medical form, you are free to be pretty creative. The oil offers many characteristics that offer delicious flavor along with the numerous health benefits they received.

You can even find them in lozenge form where you can have a long lasting flavor that provides you the relief you need. Edible CBD Oil can be found already prepared in many different flavors, even for those who may be vegan or are on a restricted nutrition plan.

Caution, however, is warranted. While they can be made into a wide variety of consumable flavors and foods, women who are pregnant, lactating, or anyone suffering from a severe illness should not consume them without consulting with a medical professional first.

Some edibles may be too strong for your system even if they do not cause psychoactive effects. The biggest advantage of using CBD edibles is that while they may take as much as two hours to take effect, they will last much longer. Whether you plan to make them yourselves or you are going to find them prepackaged for use, there is a wide selection of edibles to choose from. So, regardless of your personal preferences or needs, you should be able to find some form of edible that will work best for you.

What is Your Proper Dosage?

It is one thing to decide the type of CBD Oil you want to take in and another thing to choose the right dosage, knowing this is critical to you getting the kind of relief you need.

Unlike other medications where the label is clearly marked as to how much to take and when to take them, taking CBD Oil is not that easy. Since the results of the supplement will be based on your receptors within your body, what dosage may work for one person may not be as effective for someone else.

You also have to understand that not all CBD Oil distributors are on the up and up and may falsely represent information about the product they offer. So, determining the right CBD Oil for yourself will depend not only on the purchase but on your careful examination of the dealer you purchase from.

Start by making sure that the company you are choosing to deal with has a reputation for following the established industry standards. Check out reviews online and talk to those who have used them before. This way, you will know that the products you choose are of the best quality before you even begin.

CBD Oil is only as a good as the quality you get and the relief for your ailment will only be good if you take it in the right dosage. Take too little, and you may not get the relief you need; take too much, and you may experience some pretty negative side effects that could complicate your problem.

- Always start with the lowest possible dosage and gradually inch it upwards. This will allow the body to build up a tolerance to it and lower the risk of negative side effects.

- Unlike other drugs, your weight and body size will have little to no bearing on your tolerance level.

- When choosing capsules or oral syringes, you will be better able to control the exact dosage you need and keep that dosage consistent.

- When looking for pain relief, make sure the dosage is large enough to manage the pain and not simply just dull it.

- When treatment is for skin care, there is no usual dosage. The amount you use will be based on the type of problem you're treating and the combination of ingredients in the topical treatment.

- When choosing dosage for diabetics and blood pressure patients, it will depend on where their pancreas is in the stage of treatment. Once the pancreas begins to function normally, some stop taking insulin and then increase their dosage of CBD Oil.

Other factors that may influence your dosage could be your overall health condition. For the most part, when a person chooses to use CBD Oil, their body has already been suffering and is trying to recover from damage. This means that it may be necessary to plan for a longer treatment than would normally be needed or you may want to approach the problem more aggressively at first by choosing a larger dosage.

But if you choose to take a larger dosage at the beginning of your treatment, it is also important for you to balance it with making a few lifestyle changes. CBD Oil is considered by many to be a miracle drug, but it will always work better if your diet and habits are all working together.

Your experience in using CBD Oil should also be considered when choosing the right dosage. If you've used it before, then you are more likely to be familiar with the type of benefits you will get as well as how much you need to see results. If this is your first time using it, it is important that you learn the basic CBD Oil facts and as much as you can about the cannabis plant. This will help you be more familiar with what to expect as you begin your treatment.

We have already discussed many of these facts in this book.

- It is one of many cannabinoids

- It is non-psychoactive

- It can be taken in many forms

- Its results will be based on how it is mixed with other components of the cannabis plant or other supplemental ingredients

Even with this knowledge, we all know there is much more to be learned, and new information is being released regularly after completion of many studies of the plant and its effects on health are discovered.

CBD with THC

Sometimes, it may be necessary to use medical marijuana to treat your health issues. Some choose to escalate their treatment by using CBD Oil in addition to their standard THC. If you choose to do this, it is extremely important that you get the ratio correct. The proper ratio will depend on several different factors.

If you are treating cases of anxiety, mood disorders, or seizures, the normal ratio of 10 to 1 (CBD: THC) is recommended. However, if the treatment is for pain relief, the recommended ratio is usually more equal at 1 to 1 (CBD: THC).

If you have little experience with this type of remedy, start off with the lowest possible dosage of THC, and gradually increase it until you begin to feel that the combination is working for you.

While side effects are minimal when using hemp-based CBD Oil, you can reasonably expect to experience a few when you combine it with THC. Some complain of feeling sleepy and fatigued. This is a condition that usually appears when you first start taking it. However, resting for just a few minutes seems to help to bring the energy level back up. This condition usually fades as your body gets more accustomed to it in your system and it tends to fade within a month after beginning treatment. If the condition persists, then chances are your dosage is too high and you need to just reduce it to something your body is better able to handle.

Others worry about the risk of addiction, but it is important to understand that if you are using the purer form of CBD Oil with only a minute percentage of THC, the risk of addiction is practically non-existent. The only risk you might have is if your CBD Oil is not pure and it contains higher levels of THC than is necessary. This usually happens when you buy from disreputable dealers who have not been certified to produce quality products.

This is also the reason why you are less likely to get high. If you are purchasing quality hemp-based CBD Oil, there is not enough THC to cause you to have that euphoric high that is often associated with marijuana-based CBD Oil. This is important to know if you work for a company that requires regular drug testing as you can be confident that you won't have a risk of getting a positive result when the test comes up.

How CBD Oil is Extracted

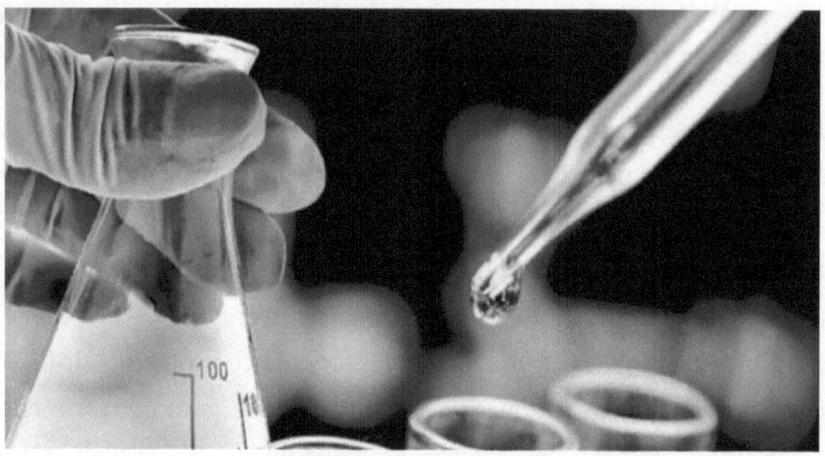

There is no question; cannabis plants have an abundant supply of CBD Oil. In fact, it is the second most abundant compound they have, making up approximately 40% of all the extracts. However, in order for it to be of good enough quality to provide the results you need, it has to be carefully extracted using very specific methods.

There are several ways to extract CBD Oil but to get the quality you need in the concentrate, there are very few extraction processes that will work the best. In order to get the most CBD from the process, the choice of cannabis variety is essential. Growers are very meticulous in choosing plant varieties that already contain a high CBD content; some even going to the extent of producing their own strains of the plant with a low content of THC to start with.

There are three primary ways of extracting CBD Oil from the cannabis.

The CO2 Method

This method forces CO_2 through the plant at very low temperatures but with high pressure at the same time. This requires very expensive equipment and can be very costly to produce. The result, however, is a high-quality oil concentrate but a very expensive end product.

The process removes unwanted substances and residue that could temper the quality of the finished product. The result is a concentrate that is a much cleaner tasting than any other form on the market.

The Solvent Method

Another highly effective way of extracting CBD Oil is by using a high-grain form of alcohol. This method, however, can destroy many of the natural oils in the process so the end product will not be as effective as an extraction using the CO_2 method. To use the solvent method, you need to have a very exacting knowledge of cannabis and the special care it takes to remove the oil.

The plant is first submerged in the alcohol-based solvents, and then the resulting solution is strained and cleaned of all solvents and plant matter. This method is extremely complicated and requires specialized training to produce high-quality oil that is marketable.

The Oil Method

Finally, the oil method involves infusing it with a carrier oil like olive oil in the process. The plant is placed in the oil of choice, which is then heated to a temperature of 100°C for 1-2 hours. This heating process extracts the CBL, which is infused into the carrier oil.

You needn't worry about loss as oil does not evaporate when heated like water would so. What you start with will be the same quantity when you finish. The drawback, however, is that the resulting oil is not as potent as the other two methods and is perishable. So once made, you will have to use it within a very short period in order to take advantage of whatever efficacy there is. Make sure that it is stored in a cold, dark place to keep its effectiveness for as long as possible.

Just in way of review, CBD is the chemical compound found in the cannabis plant. CBD Oil is a blend of natural substances that can be contained in the cannabis plant. When you produce hemp-based CBD Oil, you are actually extracting the fatty acids found in the plant's stalks. This may also contain other fat-soluble substances that also come out of the plant.

So, to put it simply, CBD oil is not pure CBD but is blended together with other beneficial substances found within the same plant. These could include fatty acids, terpenes, or some other type of cannabinoid that will help to encourage the entourage effect.

Different Types of CBD

There are also different types of CBD Oil, each with its own special effects on the body. Because CBD Oil is not pure CBD, these different types could be blended with other substances to enhance its efficacy in some way. For example, one type of CBD Oil could be used to help the body absorb it better, others may be used to make it easier to digest, and others may be used to enhance its potency.

Water Soluble Form

Basically, this type of CBD Oil is easy to dissolve in water. You will choose this form if your body is struggling to absorb medications. Many people with this problem often have to take much more than necessary just to make sure that their system can get the benefits they need. In natural science, water and oil do not blend together, making it harder for the body to absorb edible CBD. However, if you choose water-soluble

CBD, then you won't likely need to worry about that problem.

Of course, if you're planning on smoking or vaping, this won't be a problem as this is only an issue for those who choose to ingest, take it in liquid or capsule form. Still, this form is very effective and requires you to take a smaller dosage than other forms. It is also the safest and most practical because it will save you a great deal of money in the end.

Synthetic CBD

Scientists now have the ability to isolate and synthesize both THC and CBD. There are different opinions today on whether this method is good or bad. Some believe that if something is manmade, it must be harmful, yet we all know of substances within the natural environment that could kill and harm you just as easily as any chemical product produced in a factory.

Right now, your mind is probably busy conjuring up visions of mad scientists hovering over test tubes and creating some type of nefarious product that will send out evil to disrupt the natural flow of the world. However, synthetic CBD is simply a compound that is created by using a force that does not come from nature, and the result is a new compound that may not presently exist; or it can also mean creating a compound that presently does not exist in our natural environment.

We use synthetics often in everyday life. A perfect example of synthetics are the flavorings we buy to enhance the taste of our food. These are labeled as "artificial," meaning that they are specifically designed to imitate or copy the flavors that nature already offers. The advantage of these synthetics is that they are often less expensive and very close to the structure of the real deal.

So, when we stop to look at synthetic CBD Oil, we find similar benefits. Synthetic CBD Oil is not always as effective as the natural product so you will have to consume larger amounts in order to see the same results. Aside from that, they offer a host of other benefits you may not have considered.

They are less risky when it comes to increasing the dosage than the natural CBD Oil

1.   They are less expensive

2.   They have the same practical applications

There may be times when synthetics are a better option as they may carry less risk when compared to the more concentrated forms and could introduce hazards resulting from poor cultivation practices.

How to Buy CBD

We've already discussed what you need to know to choose the right dealer, but now we need to focus on how to gauge the quality of the oil itself.

We live in an age where buying any product is very easy. We simply go online, choose what we want, place an order and wait for it to come to our door. However, when it comes to buying something as important as CBD Oil, we should make sure to take extra care.

How do You Know It is Good Quality

If you are new to buying these types of products, it won't take long before you realize that all the good dealers are buried beneath thousands of questionable ones. According to some reports, less than half really do offer quality products. And when it comes to CBD, quality is extremely important for you to get the kind of results you seek.

Not to mention the fact that the oil you get may be blended with inferior products, have dangerous impurities, or have been laced with other substances that may provide more harm than good to your health.

You also need to look at the price. Unfortunately, we see many in business that inflates their prices exponentially. And while we know that CBD Oil is not cheap and that you will be shopping around for the best deals, rest assured that those who offer the lowest prices are generally not those who offer good quality.

There is expensive testing, expensive production, and even the other oils it is blended with will be costly as well. Bottom line, it is impossible to get true CBD Oil at a very low price. So, if you find a merchant offering something much lower than the average market price, it is best to assume that something is wrong and you're about to lose your money.

Because it comes in all forms, potencies, and blends, you need to know how to compare shop the right way. Some products may seem to be exactly the same but may have some underlying differences that may not be readily seen.

1.   Look at the volume: Check to see exactly how much CBD is contained in each product. Volume and quantity are not the same. The quantity is how much of the product you are getting, and the volume will tell you exactly how much CBD is contained in the product.

2.   You should notice two quantities on the label. The CBD quantity tells you the amount of CBD contained, but the hemp-oil quantity tells you the total volume of hemp-oil you are

getting. Don't get them confused; you want to be sure of the ratio of CBD to hemp-oil in every product.

3. Check the concentration. This is the amount of CBD in relation to all the other components of the product. You can find them in strengths that range from normal to a super-high strength.

4. Choose one that is best suited for your personal needs. However, if you follow two basic guidelines, you should be able to figure out which type will work best in your situation.

- Are you looking for something easy but fast?

- How much fun do you want to have?

It may sound strange to think of these questions when considering a medical supplement, but the answer to that question will immediately eliminate certain options and direct your attention to those products that will give you exactly what you need.

The only thing you will have to think about after that is how strong a dosage you need. And because there is little to no risk of getting high or having that euphoric effect from taking CBD, you can feel pretty safe in upping your dosage if you're not getting the strength you need. In essence, you're pretty much in control of your own destiny here.

Chapter 2
CBD Oil for Pain Relief

"Hemp is of first necessity to the wealth & protection of the country."

- Thomas Jefferson

Today, there is little doubt that cannabis has great healing properties, especially its two primary components, CBD and THC. While these have held wide appeal for many medical benefits, this chapter will focus on how well CBD works in dealing with pain.

CBD Oil is often used for those people who suffer from chronic painful conditions.

This has been determined based on a number of pain management studies that have shown an incredible amount of promise. It is an alternative treatment for people who are especially suffering from conditions that cause chronic pain and do not want to rely on regular medications that could either do damage to their bodies in some form or run the risk of becoming habit forming.

While much more research needs to be considered in this regard, from what we have learned so far, the oil promises to bring well-needed relief to the many people who have arthritis, migraines, fibromyalgia, back pain, IBS, neuropathy, and many more similar conditions.

How does it Work?

You could think of the receptors in your body simply as tiny little proteins that attach themselves to the cells and wait for specific chemical signals to reach them from external stimuli. The stimuli tell the cells exactly how to respond. When CBD Oil comes in contact with these receptors, it creates an anti-inflammatory reaction that can work to keep the pain level down.

According to one review conducted in 2008, which looked closely at studies performed between the years of 1980 and 2007, CBD was found to be very effective in helping patients to manage their overall pain level without any negative side effects. An additional unexpected benefit was that it was also helpful in treating long-standing cases of insomnia, which was probably a result of the pain they were suffering from.

It was found to be most helpful in patients who were suffering from multiple sclerosis. However, a more recent study, conducted in 2016, found that it was also very helpful in bringing relief to people living with arthritis. The test was conducted on rats where they applied a CBD gel for four days in a row. Afterward, they noted that there was a reduced level of inflammation and overall pain in the joints, again without the additional side effects that many people suffer from when using traditional medications.

Ingesting: This method, referred to in scientific terms as sublingual administration, is the process of placing the oil under the tongue where the substance is diffused into the blood through the softer tissues underneath the tongue. By simply dropping the oil under the tongue, it can be quickly absorbed into the bloodstream where it can be swiftly transported to the painful area providing faster relief.

Topical: The topical method works well for someone who is suffering from localized pain or pain that is the result of tension or cramps. It can come in many forms including gels, lotions, pastes, creams, lip balms, body butter, patches, scrubs, and salves.

It works well for those who are suffering from chronic arthritis, fibromyalgia, and are dealing with the type of pain usually associated with sports; perhaps the soreness you feel in the aftermath of a game, hiking, or some other type of strenuous activity.

Many have used it as a massage oil or in their bath. Some have even made them into bath bombs, or you can purchase them as bath salts already available for use.

Vaping: Another very popular form of using CBD Oil is through vaping. This works well for those who may be smokers or used to be smokers but gives them a healthier alternative to tobacco. CBD Oil has a naturally soothing effect that makes it a very appealing choice for anyone who is looking to cut down on the type of tension pain that is often associated with stress. It is not only easy to do, but it is also convenient, easy to carry with you, and can be very discreet if you know how to do it. While it doesn't offer the same flexibility as ingesting, there seems to be much more interest in vaping than there is in any other type of pain relief treatment.

There are two primary advantages you get from choosing to vape: first, it stretches out your dosage throughout the entire day. You are able to control exactly how much of it you are getting and when. Vaping is a lot easier to manage than any edible or capsule. Also, it is much faster acting and more efficient. When you vape, the oil quickly enters your bloodstream because of its ability to bypass the digestive process so you can get relief much faster than with any other method.

For anyone who is suffering from chronic pain, CBD Oil works well for helping you to not only manage the pain better but get relief from it as well. Whether you need pain relief from something related to work, or you're just suffering from a chronic condition that is slowing down your personal routine, by choosing to use CBD Oil, you will be able to easily find a wide variety of products that are not only of high-quality but available in just about any form you need. That way, you can get the help you need to ease your suffering.

When creating your CBD regimen for pain management, you must keep in mind that the best way to ensure relief is not just with a one-time dosage you take when pain occurs, but as a regular and consistent plan. This means that it must be used as a preventive form of treatment first and later altered so that you can manage flare-ups whenever they occur.

For daily management, it is recommended that you take CBD Oil on a daily basis either as a tincture or capsule form. You can start with a small dosage of 5-10mg per day. If that does not provide relief within a reasonable amount of time, then you can boost the dosage up by 5mg each time until you start of feel relief.

When the pain is located in the bones, ligaments, muscles, skin, or tendons, you could also supplement the regimen with a topical treatment like a salve or a balm. This will give an added strength to the affected area to reduce inflammation more quickly. This way, you could expect to feel relief in as little as 15 minutes and can expect it to last for several hours.

To better manage flare-ups, you can consider vaping when the pain is acute. This method brings on even faster relief as you can feel the results almost instantaneously. Of course, these guidelines are mere recommendations, and you will have to monitor your symptoms and how your body responds and adjust the treatment accordingly. This way, you will soon discover the best form of treatment for your pain and get the relief you need.

CBD Oil for Anxiety and Depression

Sometimes, we suffer from conditions that are not physical in nature, and CBD Oil can be very effective in giving us the help we need. Studies have been conducted that show the CBD oil has the ability to lower the body's automatic responses related to stress in emotional disorders as well. This is done by facilitating the neurotransmission messages in the brain and assist in performing certain neurological functions. This is why CBD has proven to be very effective in treating many cases of depression and anxiety disorders. Some of the emotional disorders that it is most effective in treating are;

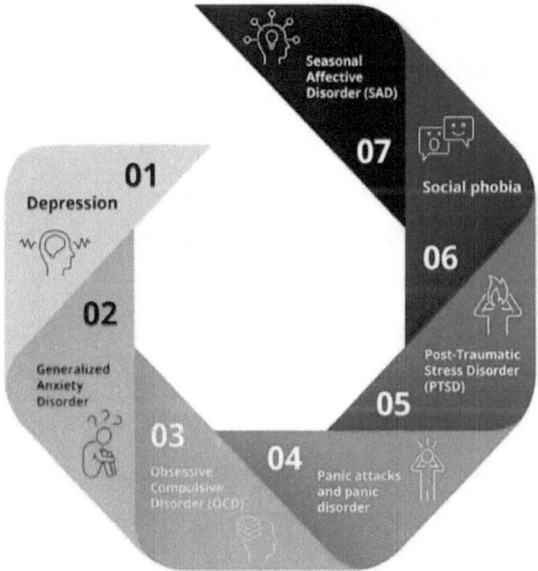

- Depression
- General Anxiety Disorder

- Obsessive Compulsive Disorder
- Panic Attacks/Panic Disorders
- Post-Traumatic Stress Disorder
- Social Phobias
- And Seasonal Affective Disorder

Sadly though, prescription medication for this type of problem can often be more debilitating than the disorder itself. They may be very effective in stopping the frequency of episodes or attacks, but they often come with very unpleasant side effects, which frequently cause feelings of apathy, oversedation, and a decrease in sex drive among other things. In essence, the side effects tend to cause more problems than the conditions themselves.

This is why CBD has proven to be a popular alternative to the harsher medications that are offered today. It is an all-natural solution that causes little to no side effects for the user to have to cope with.

After many small-scale human studies, it has been proven that CBD Oil is very effective in helping patients who are suffering from some form of social anxiety. Because of the way CBD interacts with the brain, it can quickly reduce the degree of fear, anxiety, and stress that many people have. As far back as 1982, it became evident that CBD Oil was actually very effective at counteracting THC-stimulated anxiety. While the two cannabinoids came from the same plant, the antagonism between them showed that CBD has the ability to cancel out the effects of THC.[2]

In a separate study conducted later, CBD was discovered too, under certain circumstances, lower anxiety responses in participants.

---

[2] *Dube, E. (n.d.). CBD oil and hemp oil.*

Researchers discovered that with CBD, one's brain activity was lowered in the left amygdala-hippocampus complex, the region of the brain that is most associated with conditions of depression and anxiety. The same study also revealed that there was a reduction in the participant's immediate emotional reaction to facial expressions of fear when shown.

Humans have an internal program that causes us to react to the facial expressions of other people. This is a natural and normal response we all share but, in this particular study, the reaction of the participants was considerably milder, and it lowered the chance of triggering a negative emotion when they saw someone else's negative facial expression.

While the studies conducted in this area have been limited and none of them have been extensive in their reach. The data, thus far, has shown that CBD has the ability to lower negative expressions and emotions in cases of social anxiety. The oil not only eased the levels of anxiety and any associated cognitive impairment, but it also helped to boost the participant's performance levels.

Determining the Right Dosage

When it comes to taking CBD Oil for anxiety and depression, it is important that you get the right dosage. For many, this can prove to be a real challenge because the use of CBD in this area is still very new. Since everyone is different, it will take some experimentation and a little time to get it right.

Start with the lowest possible dosage even if your specific case is severe. Don't worry if you don't see results immediately; the low dosage gives your body time to adapt to it and ensures that you are not taking more than you should. This is especially important for new users.

Gradually increase the dosage in small increments. If after taking the lower dosage, you don't begin to see results within a few days, increase the dosage in a little at a time. CBD Oil takes time to build up in the system before you see results, and its effects are often more subtle than with THC so it may take a few days before you notice any particular changes in your emotional state. So, it is imperative that you don't rush to increase the dosage until you've given it enough time to build up in your system.

Break the total dosage down to smaller ones throughout the day. Rather than taking one single dose of 500mg for the day, it is best to introduce it into your system in smaller increments. While it is safe to take CBD in large doses, taking too much at one time could cause you to lose some of its efficiency. By introducing a few drops at a time throughout the day, you give your body a chance to absorb it better and increase its efficacy at the same time.

While CBD Oil is relatively harmless on its own, it could have an effect on the potency of other medications you may be taking. You also want to make sure that your doctor is monitoring how well it is working as it may become evident that you could soon wean yourself off of the other medications you receive as your condition begins to improve. However, never take this step on your own as you will need to be monitored closely before that decision is made.

What Form of CBD Should You Take

As always, your goal is to choose the highest quality product first, then determine dosage. So, before you can decide the form, you need to find out what is available in your area and chose which products have the best quality. Then select the strength you need and then select your preferred form from what's available.

Tinctures are basically highly concentrated forms of CBD Oil and are more likely to have more medicinal properties than a simple extract, which will not prove to be as strong. This will be absorbed more slowly and will give you a much milder effect.

Because every case is different, it is imperative that you proceed with caution by starting low and building up as you go. This way, you lower your risk of developing complications or having a negative impact from taking more than is needed.

Chapter 3
CBD Oil for Cancer and Other Related Symptoms

"Why use up the forests which were centuries in the making and the mines which required ages to lay down, if we can get the equivalent of forest and mineral products in the annual growth of the hemp fields?"

- Henry Ford

To understand how CBD Oil works on cancer cells, we first need to see how cancer forms and grows. In every cell in the human body, the life of that cell is managed by a group of interconvertible sphingolipids. These hold a profile of factors called the Sphingolipid Rheostat. When a cell's endogenous ceramide (a sign that the metabolite of sphingosine-1-phosphate) is high, then the cell is about to die. If the ceramide is low, it indicates that the cell is strong and healthy.

When THC binds to the cannabinoid receptors on a cancerous cell, it creates an increase in the ceramide synthesis leading to the death of the cell. The interesting point about this is that it is believed that this only happens with cancer cells; cells that are normally healthy are not affected by the cannabinoids. The result is that it causes the cancer cells to die because it creates a tiny change in the cells' mitochondria.

The structure of most cells consists of a nucleus, hundreds or thousands of mitochondria, and an assortment of organelles contained within the cytoplasm. The mitochondria in these cells are there to generate energy for the cell to use. When the ceramide begins to accumulate, it will turn up the Sphingolipid Rheostat and as a result, increase the mitochondrial membrane pore permeability to cytochrome c, a critical protein necessary to produce energy synthesis. When this occurs, the cytochrome c is forced out of the mitochondria and killing off the cell's energy source.

The ceramide in the cancer cell also creates something called genotoxic stress on the nucleus so it can generate a protein called p53. Its role is to disrupt the metabolizing of calcium within the mitochondria. Also, it also disrupts the cellular lysosome, which the cell uses to digest nutrients needed for all cell functions. Therefore the ceramide along with other sphingolipids are actively at work to inhibit all the pathways the cancer cells need to survive, leaving it with no possible chance for it to sustain its life.

Obviously, the key here is to ensure that ceramide continues to accumulate within the cancerous cells. Based on this theory, taking in a steady amount of CBD and THC over a period of time will keep the metabolic pressure on the cancer cells so that eventually they will not be able to survive the constant onslaught.

This leads many to wonder how a simple enzyme from a plant can be so effective in fighting off such harmful physiological systems. It is primarily because our bodies are already equipped with its own endocannabinoid system that is already poised to be active by these cannabinoids.

Our own internal endocannabinoid system is already in place to protect our cells and nerves throughout the body. It allows for communication between our immune system and our central nervous system, and it is responsible for the protection of all our neurons and it micro-manages our immune system. In short, we have an internal control system that is uniquely designed to maintain our body's homeostasis and our overall health and well-being.

This is because the endocannabinoid system, while its receptors are found throughout the body, begins in the synapses of the brain. When illness or injury compromises the body in some way, it immediately calls upon the endocannabinoid system to begin coordinating the healing process. If these systems are in a weakened state, these naturally developed internal systems can be very therapeutic and instrumental in helping the body more naturally.

To better understand how this works, imagine the cannabinoid as a three-dimensional molecule. Each dimension is shaped to fit into the receptor like a key fits into a lock. We already understand that there are at least two different types of receptors, CB1 and CB2. CB1 receptors when unlocked, work to activate the CNS messaging system, and CB2, when activated, unlocks the immune system.

Both THC and CBD cannabinoids can activate both types of receptors, so they create both a neuroactive and an immunoreactive response. So, when used together to treat the type of stress, injury, or illness that demands more endogenous anandamide than the body can produce, these exocannabinoids are triggered. When the demand is sustained over a longer period of time, as in the case of cancer, then the treatment must also be sustained to maintain the pressure needed to keep the system in proper balance.

In general, CBD will always gravitate strongly towards CBD receptors located in the spleen were the heart of the body's immune system lies. From there, the cells in the immune system seek out and work to destroy the cancer cells.

After much careful research, scientists have begun to conclude that both THC and CBD do have the potential to destroy cancer cells without the need of passing through the normal immune intermediaries. In essence, these two cannabinoids are literally believed to be hijacking the pathway cancer cells used to grow and cutting off access to the enzymes it needs to survive.

While studies to confirm these conclusions are still ongoing, there is little doubt that consuming CBD Oil and THC can bring users relief from many symptoms that are commonly associated with the nasty side effects of other cancer treatments. It can help to reduce incidences of nausea, improve appetite, and help to alleviate the pain of sleep deprivation often experienced with cancer patients.

One search of the Internet will reveal thousands of claims that it is a miracle cure for such a horrific disease, however, while the studies that have been conducted show promise, they are still a long way from outright declaring CBD and THC as a confirmed anticancer agent.

According to Manuel Guzman, a biochemist in Spain, who has studied cannabis for more than two decades, many of the claims about cannabis and cancer are weak at best. However, he stops short of saying that they are outright lies. He is quick to point out that in his own studies (conducted on animals) the tumors were completely eliminated in at least a third of the subjects, and another third saw a significant reduction in size.

His reason for hesitation, he doesn't want to issue the determination before too soon. He points out that while animal studies have been very promising, the research needs to progress to the next level and include more human studies to ensure that the results will remain consistent.

Through his many years of research, he has discovered that the right combination of THC, CBD, and a drug called temozolomide have, to date, proven to be very effective in the treatment of brain tumors in mice. This cocktail seems to know exactly how to attack the cancer cells from several different ways essentially blocking their ability to spread and forcing their death.

Presently, he has started a clinical trial at St. James' University Hospital, in Leeds, England where they are treating human patients with an aggressive form of brain tumor with this cannabinoid cocktail. We are now awaiting the results, but Guzman warns against becoming overly optimistic and encourages everyone to maintain an objective position. While the evidence is clearly leaning in a positive direction, to get the studies to support his conclusions will take time, but we can be assured that in the meantime, cannabis can at least provide some relief from the symptoms and from the awful side-effects that develop from other forms of cancer treatment.

CBD Oil & PTSD

PTSD is Post Traumatic Stress Disorder, and there is no magic cure. However, if you're looking for something that can help you to manage your PTSD and function despite it, then CBD oil may be for you. Most people who have PTSD tend to self-medicate because they find it difficult to cope with the more intense and unpleasant symptoms.

People dealing with PTSD can experience hyperarousal, sleep problems, nightmares, anger and intrusive memories that impair their ability to function. Luckily, CBD oil is a way to help restore some of that power back to you. Many suitable strains of CBD will provide quick relief for people living with PTSD. It helps to get rid of the acute anxiety that

PTSD causes and promotes relaxation.

It's important to note that it will not be able to address the root of the problem. Addressing the root of the problem will require patients to seek alternative methods such as therapy, but CBD oil can help relieve symptoms fast and make the process easier. When patients are taking CBD oil, they're more likely to be in a better position when seeking other therapies and methods alongside it.

CBD Oil Treating Chronic Pain

Most pain relief medications have side effects, especially if you use them for a long time. Most pain medications are even addictive. When you become addicted to a pain killer, you'll need to continue to up your dose because it will feel like the lower doses are not working anymore. Doctors are only able to give you a handful of medication, which could leave you in a troubling situation. When over the counter drugs simply don't work, your doctor prescribes these pain relievers next including anxiety drugs, antidepressants, and muscle relaxants.

While many of these can effectively treat pain even with the possibility of becoming addict4ed, they still come with a load of other problems for most people. For some people, the side effects of this medication can be worse than the ailment you're dealing with. CBD oil is a natural alternative to the man-made chemicals that are usually prescribed. Painkillers that contain cannabinoids are often tolerated by patients very well, and they have minimal side effects they are not toxic long term either. CBD may also be combined with opioids, and in this case, the effects may be even more pronounces. There are many people in the field that believe this may be the future of painkillers.

If you're currently on pain medication that's been prescribed, talk to your doctor about adding in CBD oil to minimize the side effects of other medications that you may be taking. If you are currently taking over the counter pain medication, then you can try CBD oil before turning to your doctor to see if you need something stronger. Most people that try to use CBD oil to manage pain will not have to use other medications.

Treating Insomnia with CBD Oil

CBD oil affects the central nervous system by affecting the endocannabinoid system as well as various neurotransmitters. CBD is not intoxicating, but it does have positive effects on the mood. CBD oil can also affect serotonin receptors which regulate GABA regulators that are involved with both anxiety and insomnia.

While there are other products that you can take to help with insomnia, but once again they can have negative effects, especially when taken long term. Just as importantly, many of these medications are unnatural and can mess with the natural balance of your body. When you use CBD oil to treat insomnia, you don't have to worry about side effects. CBD oil can even help people suffering from minor imbalances in their sleep. It's best to take CBD oil for this purpose after eight pm if you plan to go to bed before or around midnight.

The only side effect worth noting is that some people will feel foggy for a little while after waking up, but this won't last throughout the day. It is not guaranteed that you'll even experience this side effect when taking CBD oil to treat insomnia. If you currently have severe insomnia, talk to your health care professional about adding CBD oil into your routine or the possibility of CBD oil replacing your current medications.[3]

---

[3] *Harris, J. (n.d.). Hemp oil & CBD.*

CBD Oil & Fibromyalgia

Fibromyalgia suffers have a hard time finding relief, but medical marijuana can help many of them. However, if medical marijuana is not legal in your state, you may want to consider turning to CBD oil instead. If you aren't aware, medical marijuana is marijuana that has been medically prescribed by a doctor in order for the patient to treat a certain illness. The National Institutes of Health says that nearly five million Americans currently have fibromyalgia, which has a variety of symptoms. These include depression, poor sleep, headaches, fatigue as well as deep tissue pain which can affect their ability to live their everyday life.

Currently, the FDA prescribes three drugs that can help to treat fibromyalgia. However, many people report that they have tried at least one if not all three of these medications and still found more help from either medical marijuana or CBD oil at treating their condition. Up to seventy percent of these patients agree that the prescriptions didn't work to give them overall relief and almost all of them experienced side effects. However, over sixty percent of the people who have tried cannabis and CBD oil to treat their symptoms found it effective, and another thirty-three said that it at least helped a little.

General Reduction in Inflammation

Chronic inflammation can cause severe issues in the body, and it can increase your risk of stroke and heart disease. Stronger bones can help to make them more resistant to inflammation as well, so it can be used proactively too!

The University of Tel Aviv did another study on rats using CBD supplements. The rats suffered from fractures, and those given CBD supplements recovered about forty percent faster than those that didn't have CBD supplements. It also provided with relief while these conditions healed. So if you're healing from a fracture or break, you can also add CBD oil into your routine to reduce inflammation, reduce pain and speed up recovery.

CBD Oil & Autoimmune Disorders

Since CBD oil can help with a large variety of autoimmune disorders too! Once again if you're having a hard time with traditional treatments and conventional medication, then CBD oil can come to the rescue. Autoimmune immune disorders can be difficult and dangerous to deal with. They often require a change in lifestyle and diet, and medication can only help so much if at all. For some people, medication causes more harm than good. Since CBD oil stabilizes your immune system and reduces inflammation, it will help with most autoimmune disorders.

You'll likely see almost immediate improvement, but it may take up to a week for some people. Even if CBD oil does not immediately help you to see larger differences, you will most likely see a reduction in swelling and pain due to these disorders. Just remember that with more severe diseases, you'll need to take CBD more often. If you are currently on a treatment method for your autoimmune disorder, you should let your doctor know before adding in CBD oil to the routine.

Treating Acne with CBD Oil

Most people already know that CBD oil is great at treating pain, but most don't know that it can help with acne too! This may not be one of the worst conditions on the list of what CBD oil can treat, but for some people, acne can be terrible. More than nine percent of the popular suffer from acne regularly, and it can be difficult to find treatment methods that actually work.

Most of the time you end up spending way too much money on a product that only helps a little bit at best. There are many reasons that you may be experiencing acne including inflammation under your skin, bacteria, genetics or overproduction of sebum. Based on recent studies, CBD oil can treat only certain types of acne, such as ones caused by inflammation under the skin. It can also help to reduce the amount of sebum that your body is producing. There was even a study that has proven CBD oil can prevent sebaceous gland cells from secreting sebum, which keeps down cytokines and other pro-acne agents.

There are different methods that you can use to treat acne using CBD oil, such as consuming it orally which is one of the most common methods, but other people have had luck with applying it topically to the area too. CBD oil also has antibacterial properties because CBD oil helps your own immune system to fight off bacteria. CBD oil has antibiotic properties, and currently, a lot of people are overusing antibiotics and have therefore become resistant to them. CBD oil is a healthy alternative, and you won't build up a tolerance to it that will cause it to become ineffective.

Using CBD Oil for Headaches

Most people who deal with headaches and have turned to CBD oil are suffering from debilitating pain. They may have even tried various medications throughout the years without seeing any large benefits from taking them. If you have regular headaches, it can impact your quality of life negatively. CBD oil will work with your brain to alleviate pain, and it can be effective for people who haven't been helped by traditional treatments. If you're currently dealing with headaches with no end in sight despite medication, then maybe CBD oil is for you.

Tension headaches can especially be treated by using CBD oil, but other headaches such as vascular migraines may also be treated using CBD oil. Vascular migraines are related to swelling of the blood vessels, and the anti-inflammatory effects of CBD oil can help with that too. If you are dealing with a headache from a nasty cold, you may find that CBD oil can help with this too as well as help you to kick that cold by boosting the immune system.

Chapter 4
CBD Benefits on Life-Threatening Diseases

"That is not a drug. It's a leaf."

- Arnold Schwarzenegger

Although CBD is still illegal in most parts of the world, it holds many benefits in the treatment and management of many life-threatening diseases, including the following:

Various Forms of Cancer

Unlike other treatments for cancer, CBD destroys tumor cells without injuring any healthy counterpart. Its treatment mechanism focuses only on the affected areas while helping to protect the unaffected counterparts. Cannabidiols also work to induce apoptosis in the glioma cells. In a study that was carried out on mice and rats, researchers found that tumor can be successfully removed using the anti-cancer and anti-tumoral qualities of CBD.

Cannabinoids play an important role in protecting normal astroglial and oligodendroglial cell lineages from the damaging effects of apoptosis mediation. When scientists McAllister and Desprez placed infected cells in a petri dish with cannabidiol, they saw how the cells stopped behaving out of control and went to their normal state upon contact with CBD.

The main reason behind these successful results is that coming into contact with CBD inhibits the overexpression of affected cells, taking away the cells' ability to grow large in size and spread to nearby and distant tissues. In turn, the affected cells get back to their original and local state so they can metastasize.

CBDs are also known for their ability to interfere with theme metastasization, adhesion, invasion, tumor neovascularization, and migration of cancer cells. The forms of cancer currently being treated with CBD are breast cancer, lung cancer, leukemia, prostate cancer, adrenal cortical cancer, endometrial cancer, testicular cancer, and uterine cancer. Aside from the studies mentioned above, numerous research-based and scientific studies demonstrate the benefits of using CBD as an anti-tumoral, anti-cancer drug.

Epilepsy and Seizure

Cannabis has a rich history as a treatment for convulsions and seizures, dating many centuries back. During the mid-19*th* century, cannabis tincture was listed in the US pharmacopeia as a remedy for pediatric epilepsy. Succeeding scientific studies claimed that the powerful anticonvulsant effects of THC, CBD, and the whole cannabis plant can help control temporal and partial lobe seizures, in terms of frequency as well as intensity. Low-THC/CBD-dominant cannabis oil extracts and strains, in particular, can facilitate significant improvement in children who have an intractable seizure disorder.

However, in a study involving children with severe epilepsy, only 10-15% of the participants who received CBD oil treatment experienced an almost complete elimination of seizures. A bigger percentage gained fair improvement (there was a reduction but not a total cessation of seizure), while some had worse seizures after taking CBD. For many parents of affected children, it takes trial and error to find the perfect concentration that suits their child. CBD oil products with low THC do not work for everyone. Therefore, all patients, regardless of age, require access to a broad spectrum of whole-plant cannabis therapies, not just high-CBD products.

CBD is showing great potential not only as a medicine for epilepsy but also for a variety of other neurological disorders. A number of experiments that were carried out in patients with neurological issues showed equally positive results. This further supports that cannabis or marijuana – despite being termed as a dangerous drug for many decades – is now being recognized as a potential cure for risky health conditions. It continues to produce remarkable results and proves itself as a reliable remedy for various life-threatening diseases.

Multiple Sclerosis

Scientists from the Cajal Institute in Madrid used cell cultures and animal models to find that cannabidiol can reverse inflammatory responses and serve as robust protection from the symptoms of multiple sclerosis. The mice that received CBD treatment for 10 days showed dramatic improvement in their condition and had excellent motor skills. Based on these findings, scientists concluded that CBD has a great ability to ease different aspects of multiple sclerosis.

Since this is a serious health condition, it is best to consult a medical specialist before inhaling CBD oil or taking any pill. Dosage and schedule of intake may vary depending on the person's situation and the type of CBD strain being prescribed. In all cases, CBD can relieve you from pain and ease the symptoms related to multiple sclerosis.

Psoriasis

Since CBD has high levels of anti-inflammatory properties, it works great against the symptoms associated with psoriasis. CBD hemp oil is naturally absorbed into the skin where it fights off inflammation to ease pain and swelling.

Besides its healing effects, CBD oil also contains antioxidants and UV protection properties, which are highly beneficial for overall skin health. And the best part is that it is a natural remedy and does not have any adverse side effects.

Diabetes

The advent of processed food and poor way of life have made people vulnerable to this kind of lifestyle disease.

Diabetes results in low levels of lipoprotein in the body and higher level of insulin resistance. Insulin resistance is a condition that disrupts the natural mechanisms of insulin, which is a hormone produced by the pancreas to help cells convert glucose to energy. In the case of type 2 diabetes, the production of insulin continues, but the cells reject to process it. In turn, the glucose builds up in the hyperglycemia and fills the bloodstream, leading to various complications.

In 2013, a study based on 5-year research revealed that CBD has positive effects on fasting insulin and insulin resistance. About half of the 4657 respondents were CBD users while the other half had never taken the drug in their lifetime. Those who were taking CBD oil reported a 17% decline in insulin resistance and a 16% reduction in fasting insulin. CBD users also had greater levels of HDL cholesterol, which is known as "good cholesterol."

In another study carried out in diabetic, non-obese mice, further development of diabetes was successfully prevented. While cannabidiol did not actually have a direct effect on glucose levels, the CBD treatment prevented the splenocytes from producing IL-12. Blocking this cytokine is essential because it plays a crucial role in the development of many autoimmune disorders.

Diabetic Retinopathy

About 80% of patients with diabetes develop another complication called diabetic retinopathy (DRP). In this condition, the retina cells are put to risk and continue to be damaged progressively. In the US, more than 12% of reported DRP cases lead to blindness.

This health condition is also linked to the breaking down of induced glucose of blood-retinal barriers. When this breakdown occurs, the neural tissues become exposed to neurotoxins, making the retina more prone to bleeding.

Obesity

Obesity, high body mass index (BMI), large waistline, and abnormal weight gain are all linked to diabetes and other related conditions. In December 2014, Obesity (journal) published a study presenting evidence that using cannabis may help reduce rates of obesity. The researchers used the Nunavik Inuit Health Survey to gather the data from 186 Inuit adults, of which 57.4% are cannabis users. They found that those who were using cannabis had:

- lower BMI, meaning they weigh less than non-cannabis users for a given height

- lower fat mass percentage

- lower level of insulin in the bloodstream when not eating; this suggests a reduced risk of developing/having prediabetes

- lower HOMA-IR or homeostasis model assessment of insulin resistance; this also suggests a reduced risk of developing/having prediabetes.

However, after controlling for the effect of BMI, researchers found no differences in both HOMA-IR and fasting insulin between non-users and cannabis users. This indicates that lower HOMA-IR and fasting insulin were not direct results of cannabis use. Rather, these were results of a lower BMI possibly influenced by the individual's habit of using cannabis.

While cannabis use does not lead directly to lower blood sugar, BMI or obesity rates, the results of the study still hold significance in terms of managing certain types of diabetes. Increasing research on CBD therapies can potentially lead to the incorporation of isolated/synthetic or whole-plant CBD use in the safe and proper management of obesity, together with regular exercise and a healthy diet.

CBD Benefits on Mental-Related Disorders

The link between marijuana and mental disorders has long been known, but for the most part, history has not been pretty. Many people claim that marijuana is an evil plant that causes people to behave abnormally and lose their right minds. However, recent medical research demonstrates how medical marijuana – with the right amount of CBD – can be useful for treating various forms of mental disorders.[4]

---

[4] *Lidicker, G. (n.d.). CBD oil: everyday secrets.*

Autism

Autism is a neuro-behavioral complex disorder that causes impairments in social language skills and communication. Its symptoms often become even more complicated due to rigid, repetitive behaviors of the patient. The severity of this condition ranges from minor limitations in speech and cognitive skills to serious impairments that require professional attention.

In the United States, 3-6 in 1000 children have autism, and the number of cases continues to increase with time. Using cannabidiol for treating symptoms of autism – such as hypersensitivity, hyperactivity, obsessive-compulsive behavior, and anxiety – has shown many positive results.

In order to effectively treat autism, medical cannabis should contain a higher amount of CBD than THC. Remember, THC causes psychoactivity; CBD does not. Dosages vary depending on the patient's specific situation, needs and lifestyle.

A study revealed that CBD also aids in regulating emotions and enhancing focus, thus is useful in preventing and treating different forms of neurological disorders. While consuming the right dosage of cannabidiol is vital for proper treatment, overdose is not a concern with this type of therapy because CBD has practically no side effects. There have been no documented cases where users died or experienced negative effects in their health. Hence, using CBD offers a sense of safety and security as a treatment for autism and other mental health concerns.

Anxiety

Social anxiety is a common form of anxiety disorder that impairs quality of life. In a study conducted in 2011, CBD showed positive effects on people with this condition who had never received any kind of treatment.

The 24 participants were grouped into two. One group was given 600mg of CBD and the other was given a placebo. The participants then underwent a simulated test for public speaking while the researchers monitored their heart rate, blood pressure, and other key signals of psychological and physiological stress. The group that received CBD showed a significant reduction in anxiety, discomfort in speech performance, and cognitive impairment; whereas the group that received placebo showed otherwise.

According to the statistics from the National Institute of Mental Health, around 15 million American adults have social phobia while roughly 6.8 million suffer from a generalized anxiety disorder. Conventional treatment typically involves medications and counseling. Using CBD as a treatment for anxiety proves to be better than antidepressants because it works quickly and does not cause withdrawal symptoms or adverse side effects.

Post-Traumatic Stress Disorder (PTSD)

People living with PTSD often become overcome with stress and anxiety, for which CBD can be an effective remedy. When ingested, cannabidiol produces anti-inflammatory and anti-anxiety effects that calm the person and slow everything down, ultimately creating a stable mental and emotional environment for the affected individual.

Since more people are accepting medical marijuana as a valid treatment option for mental conditions, it is becoming readily available in more parts of the country. CBD treatment has great potential for combatting the symptoms of PTSD, as well as easing the challenges that both the patient and family face every day.

Psychosis and Schizophrenia

Psychosis is a psychiatric term described as an abnormal state of mind, in which there is a lack of all sorts of contact with reality. It isn't a name for the disorder but a symptom of conditions like mood disorders and schizophrenia.

It is now proven that the THC content of marijuana is the culprit, not CBD. These two chemicals produce opposite effects in a user's psychiatric state, molecular signaling, and dopamine pathway.

Researchers injected CBD to rats to study its neuropathic, chemical, and behavioral effects. They found that cannabidiol alone reduces dopamine sensitization, a brain response associated with schizophrenia-related psychoses. So by using strains with high CBD and little or no THC, a person can have a tighter grip on reality.

The antipsychotic effects of cannabidiol are comparable to amisulpride, a drug commonly prescribed for psychosis. However, the former does not cause extrapyramidal side effects, higher prolactin levels, and abnormal weight gain as the latter does. CBD is also beneficial for other mental health disorders such as bipolar affective disorder.

Researchers continue to conduct major clinical trials to unearth more evidence that will prove the effectiveness and safety of using CBD oil. By then, medical practitioners may consider CBD as a primary source of treatment for different mental health issues. In all cases, consult your healthcare provider before taking any CBD-related product.

Chapter 5
Precautions and Side Effects

"The War on Drugs has been an utter failure. We need to rethink and decriminalize our marijuana laws."

- Barack Obama

Cannabidiol is generally safe for adults. It can be ingested, sprayed on the mouth, inhaled, or applied topically. But as with all forms of medication, individuals may respond differently to CBD.

Potential Side Effects

When used properly and in correct amounts, CBD does not cause adverse side effects. However, users may experience minor reactions. Some reported CBD side effects include drowsiness, lightheadedness, dry mouth, dizziness, constipation, fatigue, palpitations, teeth/mucosal discoloration, appetite change, weakness, confusion, and disorientation. Irresponsible cannabis use, especially with high THC, may lead to physical and psychological dependence.

Drug Interactions

Cannabidiol can interfere with the cytochrome P-450 enzyme system's function of metabolizing certain drugs, meaning it may increase the side effects of some medicines that are broken down or changed by the liver. The cytochrome P-450 is believed to contain over 50 enzymes that eliminate and process toxins. Following is a list of drugs that are known to use this system, thus may interact with CBD.

- Steroids

- Antihistamines

- Calcium channel blockers

- HMG CoA reductase inhibitors

- HIV antivirals

- Prokinetics

- Benzodiazepines

- Immune modulators

- Anti-arrhythmic medicines

- Antibiotics

- Anti-psychotics

- Antidepressants

- Anti-epileptics

- Anesthetics

- Beta-blockers

- PPIs

- Non-steroidal anti-inflammatory drugs (NSAIDs)

- Oral hypoglycemic agents

- Angio-tension II blockers

- Sulfonylureas

Note that the list above doesn't necessarily contain all of the drugs that could be affected by CBD. Similarly, not every drug in each of these categories will trigger an interaction. As such, you should talk to your healthcare provider before taking different medications at the same time. In most cases, dosage adjustments or alternative medications will be required. If you're worried that your cytochrome P-450 system may be malfunctioning, your physician can conduct tests to make sure that the medications you're taking are metabolizing normally.

Also, CBD may have interactions with herbs and supplements that have sedative properties, causing too much drowsiness or sleepiness. Examples of these herbs and supplements are California poppy, calamus, catnip, hops, kave, sage, melatonin, Jamaican dogwood, SAMe, sassafras, St. John's wort, skullcap, L- tryptophan, and others. CBD has no known interactions with any foods.

Precautions & Warnings

- Avoid use if you have allergic reactions or hypersensitivity to cannabinoids, peppermint oil, or propylene glycol.

- Use cautiously if you have a severe cardiovascular disease, such as ischemic heart disease, poorly managed hypertension, arrhythmias, and severe heart failure.

- Use cautiously if you or your family has a history of schizophrenia or other forms of psychosis. Correct dosing must be used.

- There is no sufficient reliable information regarding the safety of taking CBD if you're pregnant or lactating. Even so, avoid use to ensure safety.

- Some research suggests that high CBD intake might worsen tremors and muscle movement in Parkinson's disease patients. Consult your doctor before using the drug.

- Use cautiously and follow your doctor's prescription.

- Cancer patients who have urinary tract pathology may experience urinary retention.

- Avoid use if you have child-bearing potential and aren't using reliable contraception.

Proper Dosing

Concentrations in CBD products vary between preparations and may range from one up to hundreds of milligrams per dose. In order to determine a proper dosage of medications, doctors calculate the average length of time it takes for the system to process various drugs. If the system is healthy and there is only one drug to be processed, the averages are often accurate. However, drugs with the ability to influence processing times in the cytochrome P-450 enzyme system make other drugs metabolize slower or faster than they would have if taken alone. Likewise, if the system has pre-existing liver problems or other conditions, medications may not metabolize as expected.

Duration of treatment and dosages for CBD depend primarily on the person's specific needs. Since CBD oil brands follow different standards, consumers often get confused. Many brands recommend too much as one "serving" while others recommend way too little. The common serving standard for taking CBD is 25mg to be taken twice a day. It is also advisable that you increase dosage by 25mg every 3 to 4 weeks until symptoms are relieved, and decrease CBD amount if you experience worsening in any of the symptoms.[5]

Recommended Dosage for Common Conditions

For chronic pain: 2.5mg to 20mg CBD taken by mouth for 25 days on average

For epilepsy: 200mg to 300mg of CBD taken by mouth every day for up to 4 ½ months

For sleep disorders: 40mg to 160mg of CBD taken by mouth

For schizophrenia: 40mg to 1,280mg CBD taken by mouth every day for up to 4 weeks

For glaucoma: a single dose of 20mg to 40mg CBD sprayed under the tongue; note that doses higher than 40mg may increase eye pressure

For multiple sclerosis: Cannabis extracts containing 2.5mg to 120mg of CBD-THC concentration should be taken by mouth every day for 2 to 15 weeks. A cannabis mouth spray containing 2.5mg of CBD and 2.7mg of THC at doses of 2.5mg to 120mg may be taken for up to 8 weeks. Patients usually use 8 sprays within 3 hours, with 48 sprays within 24 hours, as a maximum dosage.

To increase appetite among cancer patients: 2.5mg of THC taken by mouth for 6 weeks; may be taken with or without 1mg of CBD

To ease mobility problems related to Huntington disease: 10mg of CBD taken by mouth every day for 6 weeks

Proper Usage Practices

[5] *Mindell, E. (n.d.). Healing with hemp CBD oil.*

- Take CBD medication exactly as directed.

- Use the correct spraying technique: rotate sites in your mouth between buccal locations and under your tongue.

- Store unopened CBD bottles in the refrigerator but do not freeze. You may store opened bottles at room temperature.

- Discard unused contents after 28 days and dispose properly. Do not include them in your household garbage or wastewater (e.g., in the toilet or down the drain/sink). Consult your pharmacist about proper disposal of unneeded or expired medication.

- Avoid consuming alcohol while taking CBD medications.

Consult your physician before taking additional or new medication, especially if you are trying to treat a serious medical condition.

Cannabis Extraction Methods

There are many different methods to extract cannabis—ranging from simple, DIY extractions to complex, more involved methods that are better left to the experts (HERB).

Do-it-yourself cannabis extractions are usually in the form of oil, butter, or other cannabis-infused fats. While the THC content of cannabis is practically insoluble in plain water, it is almost completely soluble in fats. When you heat cannabis in oil or butter, the THC breaks down and binds with the fat to create an easy means to introduce activated, terpene-rich addition to any dish. If you're using cannabis to improve your health, you may want to get a product with higher CBD content.

Below are three common ways to extract cannabis at home. You will need a spoon, wooden ladle, metal strainer, medium saucepan (or crockpot), and a container with a tight-fitting lid to carry out these extraction methods.

Cannabutter

Cannabutter is a main ingredient in a lot of cannabis-infused recipes. You can use it to make special space cakes or brownies, or pair it with your jam or morning toast.

Ingredients:

- ¼ oz. cannabis buds, ground

- ½ cup unsalted butter

Directions:

1. Melt the unsalted butter in the saucepan over low heat.

2. Add the cannabis grounds a small amount at a time and stir in between.

3. Simmer for 45 minutes, stirring frequently. Small bubbles should form on the surface as the blend simmers.

4. After simmering, use the metal strainer to filter out the buds as you pour the butter-cannabis mixture in the container.

5. Use the spoon to press the ground buds in the strainer and squeeze out all the cannabutter.

6. The end product will have a touch of green tinge due to cannabis. You can now use the cannabutter to make delicious cannabis-infused meals.

Canna Oil

Canna oil works great for salad dressings and sauces for snacks or baked goods. If you plan to use the oil for pasta or dressings, it's best to use an extra-virgin, fruity olive oil.

Ingredients:

- 6 cups canola oil or olive oil

- 1 oz. cannabis buds, ground, or 2 oz. trimmed leaf, ground

Directions:

1. Add oil to the double boiler or saucepan over low heat. Allow oil to heat for a few minutes.

2. Add a small amount of cannabis buds and stir until the buds are fully drenched in oil.

3. Add the remaining buds little by little until the whole amount is fused with the oil. Simmer for 45 minutes over low heat.

4. Store the canna oil in an air-tight container and keep in the refrigerator for up to two months. Discard the leftover cannabis buds in the compost.

Cannabis Coconut Oil

It can absorb more cannabinoids than other oils or butter. It is a good substitute for baked goods and can take the place of butter in many meal recipes. You may also add the oil to hot beverages for easy medication. If you choose this method, prepare to monitor the recipe for 12 to 18 hours.

Note: The amount of cannabis depends on how potent or strong you want the oil to be. Many people use up to 4 ounces of cannabis per pound of organic coconut oil. To reduce the herbal taste, soak the buds in water overnight and allow it to dry completely before grinding.

Additional equipment:

- Coffee grinder
- Thermometer
- Cheesecloth

Ingredients:

- 1 pound (16 oz.) organic, unrefined coconut oil
- 1-3 oz. dried cannabis
- Water

Directions:

1. Grind the dried cannabis in the coffee grinder until extremely fine, but not too powdery as it will be harder to filter.

2. In a crockpot, mix the coconut oil with enough water so that the oil floats in the pot. Place it over high heat and let the oil liquefy.

3. Stir the bud slowly until the oil mixture is fully saturated. Add water if needed.

4. Stick the thermometer in the crockpot and close the lid on top. Monitor the temperature till it reaches 250° F. Adjust the heat to low and continue stirring.

5. Stir periodically and make sure the temperature remains between

250 and 270 degrees. You may occasionally flip the heat setting from warm to low and back to warm to regulate the temperature.

6. The mixture should stay below 320° to keep the active ingredient from burning off. Add more water periodically throughout the extraction process so that the cannabis remains submerged.

7. After 12 to 18 hours, remove the mixture from heat and allow it to cool for a few minutes.

8. Double wrap the cheesecloth over the strainer and place it over a big container. Wrap the grounds and squeeze all the oil out.

9. Place the container in the refrigerator overnight, allowing the oil to emerge to the top. The extra water that was added in the process will catch all the remaining cannabis plant material and carcinogens from the mixture, providing a cleaner-tasting end product.

10. Take out the hardened coconut oil from the water that had sunk below. The oil will have a green color because of cannabis. Discard water.

11. Store the hardened oil in the fridge until you're ready to use it. Warm the oil before adding to your recipes.

Eating cannabis can have a different effect compared to smoking or inhaling it. For first-timers, the experience can be more intense and last much longer (if you are using a strain with high THC content). Start with adding a small amount and gradually increase it the next time until you're satisfied with the effect.

Chapter 6
Simple Cannabis Recipes

"What is weed? A plant whose virtues have not yet been discovered."

- Ralph Waldo Emerson

Once you've created your cannabutter, cannabis-coconut oil, or canna oil, you can start incorporating it to your snacks, meals, and even drinks! Here are a few simple cannabis recipes you can try.

Recipe #1 - Special Brownies
Ingredients:

- 2tbsp cannabutter

- 1 + 2 tbsp. organic, unsalted butter

- 4 oz. bittersweet chocolate

- ½ cups of cane sugar

- 1 ½ cups of white sugar

- 3 raw eggs

- 1tbsp Italian espresso, ground

- 1tbsp vanilla extract

- 1 cup of all-purpose flour

- Salt to taste

Directions:

1. Lightly grease a 13 x 9-inch brownie pan and line it with aluminum foil. Set aside.

2. Take out cannabutter, unsalted butter, and eggs.

3. Remove the chocolate from heat and add unsalted butter a little bit at a time, whisking in between.

4. Once chocolate and butter have melted, add the sugars and whisk until completely dissolved.

5. Add cannabutter, eggs, vanilla, and a pinch of salt. Whisk the mixture for 2 minutes over low heat.

6. Add the flour and mix using a spatula. Continue mixing until the flour is completely incorporated.

7. Place the batter on the greased brownie pan. Bake for 35 to 40 minutes. Avoid overbaking.

8. Cut into equal pieces and serve.

Recipe #2 - Space Cake

Ingredients:

- 1 2/3 cups of all-purpose flour

- ½ teaspoon of salt

- ½ cup cannabutter

- 1 cup of granulated sugar

- 1 ¾ teaspoons of baking powder

- ½ teaspoon of lemon extract

- ½ teaspoon of vanilla extract

- 1 cup of Crisco

- ½ cup of milk

- 2 raw eggs

- White frosting

Directions:

1. Preheat your oven to 350° F.

2. In a big bowl, mix together the baking powder, flour, and salt. Set aside.

3. In a separate bowl, combine sugar with cannabutter and Crisco. Add milk, eggs, vanilla extract, and lemon extract one at a time. Combine with the flour mixture and mix thoroughly.

4. Grease the cupcake pans and lightly flour. Then, fill the pans with cake batter about three-quarters full. Bake for one hour. Allow the cupcakes to cool before frosting.

5. Frost the space cupcakes and serve.

Recipe #3 - Cream of Cannabis Soup

Ingredients:

- 3 cups of vegetable stock

- 4tbsp cannabutter

- 1 cup of chopped broccoli florets

- ¼ cup of diced yellow onion

- 1 cup of chopped celery

- 2 cups of heavy cream

- 1 tbsp flour

Directions:

1. Pour the vegetable stock in a large pot on high heat. Bring to a boil.

2. Add broccoli and allow to cook for about 5 minutes.

3. Serve hot and enjoy!

Recipe #4 - Cannabis Tea

Ingredients:

- 1 tea bag

- 1 teaspoon of cannabutter or bud butter

- Milk (optional)

Directions:

1. Add the teabag and cannabutter/bud butter to a teacup.

2. Pour in warm or hot water.

3. Allow the butter to dissolve completely.

4. Remove the teabag and add milk if desired. Best consumed while still warm.

Nelson, X. (n.d.). *CBD Hemp Oil.*

Recipe #5 - Ganja Nachos

Ingredients:

- 3tbsp CBD oil

- 6 oz. tortilla chips

- 3tbsp light beer

- 3tbsp fresh lemon juice

- 1 cup shredded cheese

- 1 ripe avocado, cubed

- 2 garlic cloves, minced

- 1 serrano pepper or jalapeno, chopped

- 2 red tomatoes, chopped

- 1 green tomato, chopped

- 1 sweet onion, chopped

Directions:

1. Preheat the oven to 350° F.

2. Add tomatoes, jalapeno, onion, garlic, lemon juice, beer, and oil to a food processor or blender. Pulse three times to make the texture chunky.

3. Spread the tortilla chips on the baking sheet and cover with shredded cheese. Top with a heaping spoonful of the blend you just prepared.

4. Top with avocado cubes and serve.

Recipe #6 - Ganja Garlic Bread

Ingredients:

- 1 16oz loaf of French bread or Italian bread

- 1 stick (1/2 cup) softened cannabutter

- 2 large garlic cloves, minced

- 1tbsp parsley, freshly chopped

- ¼ cup Parmesan cheese, grated

Directions:

1. Preheat oven to 350° F.

2. Cut the Italian/French bread horizontally in half. In a bowl, mix garlic, parsley, and cannabutter together and spread the mixture over the bread.

3. Place the buttered bread on a baking pan and heat for 10 minutes in the oven.

4. Take out the pan and sprinkle grated Parmesan cheese over the bread. Put it back in the oven and broil for 2 to 3 minutes on high heat, until the cheese bubbles and the bread edges start to toast. Monitor the bread closely to prevent it from getting burnt.

Recipe #7 - Canna Oil Infused Guacamole

Ingredients:

- 2 ripe avocados

- 4 teaspoons of canna oil

- 1 tomato, chopped

- ½ teaspoon of kosher salt

- ¼ cup of cilantro leaves, finely chopped

- ½ red onion, cubed

- 2 fresh medium limes

Directions:

1. Mash the avocadoes in a bowl and add all the remaining ingredients.

2. Mix thoroughly until everything is completely incorporated.

Tip: Drizzle in citrus juice onto the guacamole and press a plastic wrap tightly into its surface to keep it from turning brown. This technique limits oxygen exposure that causes browning.

Chapter 7
What about Side Effects?

"Hemp is going to be the fiber of choice in both the home furnishings and fashion industries."

- Calvin Klein, 1997

Under most conditions, people report that there are no side effects of using CBD oil. However, there is always the rare case, which we'll talk about in this chapter. Though, you'll find that most CBD oil side effects are relatively minor. There are two main side effects that people experience when taking CBD oil. Just keep in mind that side effects are never the same for everyone. Some people will just experience mild to no side effects, but others may find them to be more severe.

Light Headedness

Lightheadedness isn't unheard of when using CBD oil, but it luckily isn't a common side effect either. It is often due to low blood pressure. When you take too much CBD oil, you can lower your blood pressure. If this is going to be a side effect you experience, you'll likely see the results within twenty minutes to an hour after taking your dose. This is just temporary, and if you're taking medication for your blood pressure, always stick to the recommended dose of CBD and start slow. Stevens, R. (n.d.). *CBD oil for pain relief.*

Fatigue

Once again, this is an uncommon side effect of using CBD oil. For the most part, CBD oil will produce the opposite result. If you experience fatigue, it's likely because your dose is too high which can cause drowsiness. If you are taking the proper dose of CBD oil, then you should feel that you've been filled with energy and have the ability to concentrate.

Stevens, R. (n.d.). *CBD oil for pain relief.*

Chapter 8
A Deeper Look at any THC Content

"To connect with this miracle.....Choose for divine flow, divine balance, all in divine order. It's given to you according to your belief."

- Mom

We've previously talked about how THC is a psychoactive compound, which is where the high comes from cannabis. CBD oil has to have 0.3% or less THC in it to be legal. This will go undetected in your body, which means it isn't enough to get you high. However, small doses of THC with CBD oil can help with some ailments. It will depend on if THC is legal in your state. If it is legal recreationally, then you have nothing to worry about. If it is legal medically, then you may want to talk to your doctor about using it to address any medical conditions that you have. Certain strains have been crossbred to have the qualities it needs to treat certain illnesses.

We've already discussed that CBD oil that has higher THC will better treat epilepsy and seizures. Just remember that if it is not legal in your area, then you are breaking the law. Penalties for breaking the law are often harsh and don't care about your intentions. Always remember that some conditions can be treated with CBD oil, but only with a higher content than legally allowed.

When You'll Need Higher THC

Here are a few times you may need a higher THC level to reap the full benefits of CBD oil.

- Increasing the appetite of cancer patients.

- Treating Chronic Pain for some Patients

- Managing Epilepsy and Seizures

- Symptoms of Huntington's Disease

- Treating Severe Sleep Disorders, such as extreme Insomnia

- Helping with Multiple Sclerosis

- Helping to Treat Schizophrenia in Some patients

- Treating Glaucoma

CBD Oil as a Concentrate

As the name suggests, a CBD oil concentrate is the strongest dose of CBD you can take. Compared to other CBD products, this is the higher concentration and there is no dispute. It's convenient if you have to take a higher dose of CBD oil for any condition that you're treating.

Keep in mind that CBD concentrate is usually not flavored, and the natural flavor of this oil is intensified, which makes it less tasty for others. CBD concentrates are popular due to their easy quick dosage and high potency. Just put it along the cheeks and tongue, and let it dissolve. You'll find it very similar to the tincture method. It will last about three hours, but it may take up to fifteen minutes for a CBD concentrate to kick in.

CBD Oil as a Tincture

Tinctures are one of the purest forms that you can use CBD oil in. There is no extra processing to the oil, but some brands do offer flavorings. That choice is completely up to you. Flavoring will make CBD oil a little easier for people to take because it will mask the unique taste, but it won't affect the purity of your product. Without any flavoring, CBD oil as a nutty and earthy taste which some people don't find unpleasant.

Taking a tincture is easy! CBD oil can also stain clothing or furniture depending on the material that it's made of.

Tinctures are more effective and you can prevent straight away swelling. You can instead ingest as much of it as you can sub-bilingually. This means you'll want to place a few drops along the cheeks or alternatively under your tongue. Just leave them there without swallowing for a little while so that the CBD can absorb into your bloodstream before going into your digestive tract. If you use this method, you'll notice some effects within ten to fifteen minutes, and these effects typically last around there hours. Just for reference, if you get a 30 ml tincture, then you'll get about 720 drops out of it.

CBD Oil as a Topical Treatment

It's more and more common for CBD oil to be in topical applications such as lotions, lip balms and salves. They're perfect for anti-aging, and as discussed previously, it can even help to treat acne, inflammation, chronic pain, psoriasis and, of course, treat wrinkles. When you're picking out a topical product, you should look for words such as encapsulation, Nano-technology or micellization. This will prove that the CBD product can carry it through dermal layers which will provide you with relief.

If you're using something infused with CBD, you'll use them like you would any other care product. Only use it as necessary, and you will apply it directly to the area. Of course, make sure the application is generous, and make sure to rub it in without being too harsh on an area that is hurting. Small, slow circles usually are best to massage the area and make sure none of your product is wasted. It can take fifteen minutes for a topical treatment of CBD oil to take effect, but it'll last just as long as ingesting CBD oil. Later in this book, you'll learn how to add CBD oil to various salves and creams to make products that can help you to achieve the same effect.

CBD Oil as a Spray

This will have the weakest concentration of CBD oil, so most users will stay away from this. You'll typically find CBD sprays to contain one to three milligrams, which is considerably low when you compare it to other products. Also, sprays can be inconsistent, so it isn't recommended nearly as well. The reason people may choose a spray is that it's easy to carry around, especially if you travel. If you're traveling, taking the spray on the road is easier and you're less likely to spill something like a tincture or concentrate.

If you're using a spray, you may need to use it on the area a few times before you notice any effects due to the concertation. Sprays are often taken orally, and you spray them straight into your mouth. However, each spray is different so always check the label. You don't want to ingest a topical spray accidentally! The serving size per use will be two to three sprays. If you're using a spray, you may want to use it with CBD capsules as well. It will top of the concentration and make it easier if you need a pick me up in the middle of the day. Sprays will typically kick in within ten minutes, but they last considerably less time than other methods.

Sprays will only last for one to two hours.

Vaping with CBD Oil

Most people know what vaping is by now, a type of smoking using a vape pen which does not contain nicotine. What most people don't know is that you can vape with CBD oil. If you like vaping, then this may be a method that you want to try. If you don't, then there's no reason to start. It's no more concentrated than any other type of CBD oil product. Actually, vaping has been reported to have lower effects compared to other methods. Remember that concentrate is the highest dose of CBD oil you'll find.

Though, if you're worried about drawbacks, vaping can be an easy solution. It's considered a convenient and relaxing way to take CBD oil orally without having to worry about the taste. You will find naturally flavored CBD as well as flavored cartridges. Once again, it'll kick in after about ten minutes. Sadly, just like with CBD oil sprays, it will only last one to two hours.

CBD Oil as an Edible

CBD oil as a vape, may not be great for some people. Instead, you may want to try an edible. It can be harder to get ahold, making it one of the least favored ways to take CBD oil. However, you may need more relief than a topical solution may be able to provide you with much-needed relief. If you are hoping to try something a bit different, then check them out. It's a great option if you're using CBD oil in the long term. It can be worthwhile to mix up the routine from time to time edibles are a great way to do that.

So what is edible CBD oil? It's a food or beverage that contains CBD oil.

Of course, you can add CBD oil to any snack or meal you make, and many people do use CBD oil in a smoothie, but edibles are typically something you buy. Of course, you can add it to breakfast, snacks, or any drink! If you don't like the taste, just try it out! You just need to remember that when you use CBD oil as an edible, it can take longer for it to kick in.

CBD Oil as a Capsule

CBD oil can also be taken as a capsule for those who simply hate the taste of the supplement. For some people, it's even easier to use because they can just take it with their normal vitamin. If you're already taking a supplement or medication on a daily basis, then CBD pills may be the way to go. The amount that you take will depend on the capsule you get, which could be between 10 mg and 25 mg of CBD per pill. Each capsule is already filled, so you have a clear set amount that you'll be taking, making it easier to monitor your dose.

Sadly, if you want to change doses, it can be hard if you're taking pills. You can't just cut a capsule in half since they're full of liquid. While you're still trying to determine what dose to take, you should use another form of CBD oil. Once you know exactly how much to take, then you can more easily switch to a capsule. If you're hoping to scale your dose up, you can easily take a capsule along with other CBD products including tinctures so that you can adjust your dose or add in a smaller dose during the day after taking your capsule. When you take a capsule, remember to stay hydrated to get the desired result. When you take capsules, it can take anywhere between a half hour to two hours for them to really kick in since capsules have to be broken down by your digestive tract. Like most CBD products, the effects can last up to four hours.

Finding the Right Dosage

Dosage is a difficult thing to pinpoint for most people. It's a gray area that requires experimentation to get it right because everyone reacts to CBD oil a little bit differently. Only Hemp oil manufacturers can sell CBD oil as a supplement. No current data tells a person exactly how much they should be taking depending on their weight, age and condition like most medication. As CBD oil becomes more popular, the research about CBD oil also increased. Companies want to educate you and convince you're of how CBD oil can help you.

Almost everyone can benefit from CBD oil, but how much you should take to benefit is still in question. Since CBD products are required to add serving size and nutritional information on their food labels, you shouldn't use these labels to tell you how much to take. The servicing size on these labels is more of an educated guess that may not immediately work for you. Currently, there are no real negative side effects from taking too much other than the two mentioned previously, which can easily be remedied by scaling down your dose.

So what is recommended? Keeping a journal is always beneficial, but more so you'll need to look at your bodyweight to figure out where to start.

Think about what you're taking CBD oil for. If you want to take it for your general health, then start by taking 2.5 mg and scale up to 15 mg if needed. If you're treating yourself for nausea while going through chemotherapy, then consider taking upwards of 30 mg every day. If you're dealing with chronic pain, then try up to 15 mg a day. If you're dealing with a severe sleeping disorder, you may even need to take 40 to 160 mg, but this will depend on your weight. If you are heavier, such as over 200 lbs., then you'll want to take it on the higher side. If you don't weigh that much, then you'll want to stick to the lower dosage.

About CBD Strains

CBD oil isn't just CBD oil. There are different strains to consider, and yes some are more potent than others. They also have different levels of THC. Some will work differently toward symptoms depending on the chemicals in that particular strain. There have been many that are crossbreed to create a specific plant that has specific effects and qualities. Of course, more types will crop up as CBD becomes more popular and more scientific studies are conducted. In this chapter, we'll go over some of the most popular strains and what makes them different.

Charlotte's Web

This is great if you're looking to treat seizures. The THC content is 0.3%, so it has a high CBD content which was cultivated by the Stanley Brothers, and it was specifically made to help epileptic patients. Of course, it's become more popular recently. With this strain, you may feel dizzy when you first start your dosage, but your body should adjust.

Harlequin

This is a Sativa dominant type of CBD strain. It comes from a few different types of plants including Colombian Gold, Nepali Indicia, Swiss Landrace and Thai. However, it has a 5:2 ratio of CBD to THC, so you should make sure it's legal in your area. It's great for treating moderate pain and anxiety, and it has a unique flavor that many people find easier to take. It won't make you feel drowsy, but it will take care of most pain.

Cannatonic

This strain comes all the way from Spain, and the THC is below six percent. It has a high CBD content that is above seventeen percent, and it's another crossbreed. It's between a male G13 Haze and a female MK Ultra. G13 Haze is mostly a medical strain that helps with pain, migraines, anxiety as well as muscle spasms. This has the best of both!

Pennywise

This is a 1:1 ratio, so once again it may not be legal in your area. However, it's extremely helpful with treating depression or anxiety if it is legal in your area.

MK Ultra

This is a cross between OG Kush and G-13. T.H. Seeds bred it, and it's quite unique. It has a hypnotic effect, which helps it to get into your system pretty quickly. It's considered to be a strong stain that will last long in your system. You should use this much more sparingly.

Sour Tsunami

The CBD in this is higher than the THC, so it may be legal in your area. It's great if you're trying to treat chronic inflammation or pain resulting from inflammation. You won't find any unwanted side effects, and the CBD is up to ten percent. It's a Sour Diesel and NYC Diesel cross, which has a musky smell. However, it does have sweet undertones.

Canna-Tsu

This is a balanced THC/CBD strain, so it isn't legal unless you have a medical marijuana card for your state or are in a state where recreational marijuana is legal. It has a distinctive and unique smell that's earthy, sweet and has a touch of citrus. It's great if you are looking for the mental benefits of CBD oil. This particular strain promotes a feeling of wellness.

Colombian Gold

This strain is also for anxiety, but it will also help concentration and focus. It's great for treating muscle tension as well as mild pain. The user will usually feel happier as well as alert. This is a unique strain that can also treat ADHD/ADD.

ACDC

This is a CBD dominant strain, where it's 20:1. There is very little THC, but it's a great option for those who are trying to treat anxiety since ACDC reduces stress, which also helps with depression. Due to the ratio, it's great for relieving pain and tension as well. Of course, this strain is only for mild to moderate pain.

Sour Diesel

This strain is also nicknamed "Sour D". It will help to give you the energy you need so that you're alert and focused. It's perfect for treating stress or depression. It helps with anxiety, and it can help with pain. It also has the added benefit of lasting in your system for a long time compared to other strains, which is perfect if you have to take CBD oil regularly.

Conclusion

Thanks so much for buying this book. Now that you learned that it is possible to experience natural relief without the high using CBD hemp oil and more importantly, how to use it properly, I would like to strongly encourage you to act on what you've learned here. Why? Knowing is just half the battle for relief and the other half is action. Take the first step of consulting a medical professional or a legit marijuana expert. If you can't find one, ask the store where you plan to get your first bottle of CBD hemp oil about the appropriate dosage for the condition you'd like to treat and legalities of purchasing and using CBD oil in your area. Also, start with the lowest dosage first. That way, you can optimize the relief and other health benefits CBD hemp oil can provide. The longer you put action off, the higher the chances you won't do anything. And with that, your chances of experiencing natural relief without the high become lower and lower.

Finally, always keep in mind that CBD hemp oil isn't considered as prescription medicines anywhere in the world. As such, you should give it a shot with the mindset that it may, or it may not work. However, studies and anecdotal evidence show the promising relief and health benefits of CBD hemp oil. Because of that, you can be hopeful that there's a very good chance that you may experience relief – and other potential health benefits - without the high through CBD hemp oil.[6]

---

[6] Rosenthal, T. (n.d.). CBD hemp oil 101.

Check Out Our Other Books:

1. Resolving Anxiety and Panic Attacks

A Guide to Overcoming Severe Anxiety, Controlling Panic Attacks and Reclaiming Your Life Again

Worldwide, one in six people is affected by a mental health disorder. So you are not alone in this (Ritchie & Roser, 2019). There is a difference between clinical anxiety and everyday anxiety. Everyday anxiety is normal and in often cases, it is necessary, while chronic anxiety will leave you functionally impaired. This book will not only inform you about anxiety and panic attacks but also introduce you to various methods and techniques that aid in getting rid of anxiety. It is a perfect package if you want to make long-lasting, meaningful changes in your life in a way that gets rid of anxiety. Knowledge is power, so gaining information about anxiety and panic attacks already puts you in the lead against them.

In the first chapter, we'll start with the basic knowledge of panic attacks and anxiety. The symptoms of both are pretty much the same, but there are some major differences as well. Knowing their difference and similarities can help you clearly understand your condition. Some basic ways of coping with them are also explained alongside their symptoms.

After gaining knowledge about anxiety and panic attacks in the first section, you will seek answers and ways to overcome them. The second chapter goes more in detail about the physical effects of anxiety. There are some types of anxiety which are also talked briefly about in the chapter. There are also therapies and treatments that are used to overcome and control anxiety. Their details are discussed in the chapter from where you can figure out what sort of treatment will suit you better. Some other ways of coping with anxiety are also discussed and they will surely prove beneficial to the reader.

The third chapter will make you aware of how interrelated physical and mental healths are. There are also details on how to improve one's physical health to influence a person's anxiety positively. You will also learn how important practicing well-being is. If you are to ignore physical health, it will cause problems for your mental health as well.

The fourth chapter will delve deep into mindfulness and its vast benefits. Mindfulness is a very powerful tool we have but don't know how to use. It can be practiced through meditation techniques, etc. It makes us see things more clearly than ever before. Practicing Mindfulness will arm you against any anxiety and panic attacks. In this chapter, it is explained in detail what it means and what are its advantages.

In the fifth chapter, we will learn about meditation and how can it help manage anxiety. We first start off by knowing what it is. You also have got to know its benefits and various techniques from which one can pick according to their choice. We will also learn the accurate posture you should have during meditation. We will learn how mediation reinforces our brain to stave off anxiety and panic attacks. It is a long road but a successful one for sure. Besides helping us out with anxiety and panic disorder, meditation has numerous other benefits for our body and mind.

The sixth chapter will explore the meaning behind self-love and its importance in fighting anxiety. Our battle with anxiety has to start from a positive ground. We first have to be fully comfortable and respectful towards ourselves. You will also find out how lack of self-love can actually breed anxiety.

Opening about anxiety is not an easy task but could be very helpful against anxiety. How to go about the whole process is talked about in detail in the seventh chapter. You will also learn how to evaluate your therapist and choose the right one. In this chapter, there are also guidelines for people who have just recently become aware of their anxiety and now they want to seek help. It will give them knowledge about things to consider when talking to someone about mental health, what you should accept and be prepared for. There is also information about talk therapy there.

In the eighth chapter, we address the misunderstanding about anxiety. Despite affecting so many people, it remains a different experience for all of them. There are also common mistakes pointed out in that chapter which we'll go into detail the mistakes that make our anxiety worse.

The ninth chapter is about where we talk about putting our foot down and start to incorporate practices into our life which will help you get rid of anxiety and panic attacks. We will learn how to manage our responses. It is basically a comprehensive listing of all the things you should be avoiding or adapting to lead a healthy lifestyle free of anxiety.

*Want to read more? Purchase our book on **Anxiety and Panic Attacks** today!*

2. Cognitive Behavioral Therapy

How CBT Can Be Used to Rewire Your Brain, Stop Anxiety, and Overcome Depression

Cognitive stems from cognition, which encapsulates the idea of how we learn and the knowledge that we carry. The things you learn are part of your cognition, and what you do with that information is included in that category as well. Cognition includes a wide list of information that you might not fully realize.

Behavior is what we do. It is how we act. The things that you choose to say to other people are all about your behavior. How you react to what others have to say will exhibit your behavior as well. Your behavior is all about your mind interacting with your body and how that interacts with the people and other things that surround you.

Therapy is any form of help, usually from a trained professional, to help improve on whatever the therapy is specified for. You might get physical therapy to help regain strength in your knee after having a serious surgery. You can also get therapy to help overcome an alcohol or drug addiction.

Throughout this book, we're going to give you the basis you need to start understanding cognitive behavioral therapy. The three together—cognitive, behavioral, therapy—all make up CBT, which is a method that is going to directly help you overcome the mental illness that you are hoping to treat.

Therapy can be expensive, and even if you do have the means to go through with this process, you might struggle to find the right therapist. Sometimes, you might live in an area where there is only one therapist within a close distance, but you don't have a vibe with them that you find to be helpful. You might also find that you are desperate for help and that you want a therapist, but insurance coverage isn't always good for this.

By reading this book, you'll be able to find the tools you need to help with overcoming your most challenging thoughts. We are going to take you through the steps to identify the root issues and come up with specific methods to get you through.

Want to read more? Purchase our book on **Cognitive Behavioral Therapy** *today!*

3. Effective Guide On How to Sleep Well Everyday

The Easy Method For Better Sleep, Insomnia And Chronic Sleep Problems

"A well spent day brings happy sleep." — Leonardo da Vinci

Are you experiencing the worst restless feeling? Has your doctor diagnosed you with insomnia, restlessness, sleeplessness? When the whole world around you seems to be in peaceful deep slumber, you are the one who is restless. No matter what term is used to describe it, the fact is that it is you who is actually going through insomnia, and nothing could feel worse than that.

So you drag yourself from bed in the morning feeling as earth, with its entire lock stock and barrel, has decided to perch on your head for the day. Yet you go through the motions of the day, though you barely manage to make it through the hours. By the early night, you fall on to bed hoping this night will be different because you're dead tired and nothing will keep you from sleeping like a log. It's 2.00 a.m. now, dawn is breaking through and there you are, still wide awake and ready to scream to the world because no matter how tired you are or how hard you have tried, you simply can't get to sleep.

While there are proven facts and evidence of the devastating effects of sleeping less, the investigations are still on to establish the exact nature of effects resulting from too much sleep. Some researchers argue that people who sleep much longer than necessarily have a higher death rate. Physical and mental conditions such as depression or socioeconomic status can also lead to excessive sleep. There are other researchers who argue that the human body will naturally restrain it from sleeping more hours than really necessary. However, with research still underway for concrete evidence of the effects of over sleeping the best path you can choose is to adopt a sleeping pattern somewhere in the middle. According to the National Sleep Foundation, this middle range falls between seven and eight hours of sleep during the night. Despite these statistics, the best way to ensure you receive sufficient sleeping time is to let your own body act as your guide. You can always sleep a little extra if you feel exhausted or sleep a little less than usual if you feel you are oversleeping.

Dangers of Sleep deprivation.

Though sleep is something the average human being takes for granted, it is also one of the greatest mysteries in life. Just like we still don't have all the answers to the quantum field or gravity, researchers are still exploring the reasons behind the 'whats' and 'whys' of sleep. However, one fact unchallenged about sleep is that a proper sleep is paramount for maintaining good health. The general guideline regarding the optimal amount of sleep for an adult range from six to eight hours! If you carry on with too little or too much of this general guideline you are exposing yourself to the risk of adverse health effects.

Though sleep is something that comes naturally to many people, the problems of sleep deprivation have today become a pressing problem with more and more people succumbing to chronic sleeping disorders. Unfortunately, a great number of these people do not even realize that lack of sleep or sleep deprivation is at the root of their manifold problems in life. Scientific research also points out that lack of sleep on a continuous scale can lead to severe repercussions on your health.

If you have been experiencing impaired sleep patterns for a longer period, you also face the risk of:

- Severely impairing your immunity strength

- Promoting the risk of tumor growth, as it has been scientifically established that a tumor can grow at least two to three times faster among animals subjected to severe sleeping dysfunctions within a laboratory setting.

- Creating a pre-diabetic condition in the body. Insomnia creates hunger, making you want to eat even when you have already had a meal. This situation can lead to problems of obesity in turn.

- Critically impairing memory. How many times during the day have you found it difficult to remember even the most mundane and repetitive events when you have had no more than 4 – 5 hours of sleep? Even a single night of impaired sleep plays havoc with our memory faculties, just think what it can do to your brain if you consistently lose sleep.

- Ruining your performance level both physically and mentally as your problem-solving abilities will not be working in peak order.

- Stomach ulcers

- Constipation, hemorrhoids

- Heart diseases

- Depression, lethargy and other mood disorders

- Daytime drowsiness

- Irritability

- Low energy

- Low mental clarity

- Reaction time slows down

- Lower productivity

- More accidents and mistakes

- Lower levels of growth hormone and testosterone

The growth hormone in the body which is vital for maintaining our looks, energy, and skin texture is produced by the pituitary gland. The specialty of this hormone production procedure is that it is only produced during the times of deep slumber or during intense workout sessions. In the absence of normal production of the growth hormone, our bodies will start on a premature aging process. According to research, people suffering from chronic insomnia are three times more susceptible to contract fatal diseases. When you lose sleep overnight, you cannot make up for it by sleeping more the next day. A night's lost sleep will be lost forever. More alarmingly if you continue to lose sleep regularly, they will create a cumulative negative effect that will disrupt your general health. All in all, sleeping deficiencies can effectively make your life miserable, as you already know.

How Much Sleep Do I Really Need?

This is a question that remains a mystery just like the questions of why and what makes us want to sleep. In response to a question of how many hours of sleep do we really need, an expert has answered that it is actually lot less than what we have been taught. On the other hand, though a good night's sleep is vital for good health, overdoing the sleeping can be equally bad for us. But if you sleep less and continue this for too long, the result will be confusion between body and brain signals, resulting in muddled thoughts, lethargic feelings, and overall lassitude. So, the question remains, how many hours of sleep do we really need? Is it essential to sleep the prescribed number of eight hours a day or is catching up a good sleep on a five to six-hour basis enough?

The eight hours of sleep theory is increasingly becoming unpractical in this fast-paced lifestyle. Actually, the recommendation of eight hours of sleep arises based on the idea that our ancestors had their beauty sleep between 8-9 hours in the past. In today's context, this concept is regarded more or less as a myth. In a study conducted by the Sleep Research Center, youngsters within the age group of 8 to 17 generally sleep for about nine hours during the night. However, in the case of adults, this theory is not applicable as a majority of them are sleepless and many of them thrive after a solid sleep varying between 5-7 hours.

A research conducted by the National Institute of Health has established that people who sleep soundly for nine hours a day or more are actually two times more vulnerable than those who sleep less in developing

Parkinson's disease. A study report released by the Diabetes Care states that people claiming to sleep less than five hours or more than nine hours daily are the ones with the highest risk of attracting diabetes. In contrast, a large number of contemporary studies prove that people with sleeping patterns that do not exceed or fall beyond seven hours daily possess the highest survival rate. The persons who experience sleeping disorders and sleep less than 4.5 hours have the worst survival rate.

When ascertaining the correct number of hours you should sleep, the fact is that there is no magic number of hours. It will depend on a person to person basis as well as factors like age, activity, and performance level. For example, smaller children and teenagers require more sleep compared to adults. Your personal requirements will not be the same as your friend or colleague who is of the same age and gender as you. Because your sleep needs are unique and individual. According to the National Sleep Foundation, the difference of sleep requirements between two people of the same age, gender, and activity level is due to their basal sleep needs and sleep debt.

Your basal sleep need is the number of hours of sleep you typically need to engage in optimal performance levels. The sleep debt comprises of the accumulated number of hours of sleep you have lost as a result of poor sleeping habits, a recent sickness, social demands, environmental factors, etc. A healthy adult generally possesses a basal sleep need between seven and eight hours each night. If you have experienced sleeping difficulties and as a result accumulated a sleep debt you will find that your performance level is not up to its usual standard, even if you wake up after seven or eight hours of restful sleep. The symptoms will be most apparent during the times the circadian rhythm naturally alters like during mid-afternoon or overnight. One of the ways of easing out of an accumulated sleep debt situation is to get a few extra hours of sleep for a couple of nights until you regain your natural sleeping rhythm and vitality during the day.

Understand what Kind of a Sleeper Are You?

Sleep, dear reader, is the precious restorative that rights so many physical and mental wrongs. The elixir that transforms life and puts a spring in your step, a smile on your face, and the feeling that you can take care of everything that comes your way is sleep. Undervalued, ignored, and forgotten until you wake up to the realization that it's one of the essential foundations of daily wellbeing.

So what kind of a sleeper are you? There are many studies and descriptions of how we sleep but the common consensus settles for the following five simple categories:

1. Lively, healthy early risers!

These happy individuals usually get the sleep they need and rarely feel exhausted or fatigued. They are typically younger than the other groups, usually married or with a long-term partner, working full-time and definitely a morning person with no serious medical conditions.

2. Relaxed and retired seniors.

This is the oldest group in the survey with half of the sample being 65 or older. They sleep the most with an average of 7.3 hours per night compared to 6.8 across all groups. Sleep disorders are rare even though there is a significant proportion with at least one medical disorder.

3. Dozing drones.

These busy people are usually married/partnered and employed but they often work much longer than forty hours a week. Frequently working up to the hour when they go to bed, they get up early so they're always short of sleep and struggle to keep up with the daily pressures of life. Statistically, they'll feel tired or fatigued at least three days a week.

4. Galley slaves.

This group works the longest hours and often suffers from weight problems as well as an unhealthy reliance on caffeine to get through the day. Shift workers often fall into this group and there is also a marked tendency to be a night owl or evening person. They get the least amount of sleep and are more likely to take naps yet, surprisingly, this group often believes that, despite the state of their health, they are getting enough sleep.

5. Insomniacs.

Here is the largest proportion of night people and many of them quite rightly believe they have a sleep problem. About half of this group feels they get less sleep than they need and the same proportion admits to feeling tired, fatigued and lacking energy most of the time.

So, which of the five groups do you think you fit into?

If you're a happy member of Group One, your sleep should by definition be absolutely fine. Don't worry. We've got some really good ideas to share with you to keep you right on track and we'll even add some special extra features to your nightly rest routine to maximize the experience. If you're not in this group, our aim is to help you become a full-time member of the healthy, happy sleepers' association! Membership is for life.

Group Three represents too many tired, irritable, and generally inefficient individuals whose quality of life is impaired because they're too tired too often. Their work suffers because they rarely have sufficient rest to successfully assimilate the day's events. Their home life is degraded because work intrudes too often and they're just too tired to enjoy the pleasures and comfort of a life away from work. Feeling tired becomes their default position and they know they need to do something to give their minds and bodies the rest they deserve. Individuals in this group frequently suffer from long- term mental, physical and emotional stress.

The fourth group is rightly described as the night owls. They work the longest hours and, as we noted above, they typically work shifts. The health problems associated with this group include a marked tendency towards obesity as well as a range of inflammatory diseases. Despite the fact that these people rarely look or feel well, they seem to ignore the evidence and usually claim to get enough sleep, relying on sugary energy drinks and caffeine to keep them awake during waking hours. They take naps because their bodies can't function without additional sleep during the day. An objective analysis of their health would typically reveal a range of health and wellbeing issues.

Insomniacs are the dominant members of Group Five, people who don't get enough sleep, can't get to sleep, and who know they have a problem. Unfortunately, many insomniacs end up taking prescription medication to deal with their symptoms and we have to question the benefits of this solution in light of the many unpleasant side effects associated with long-term sleeping pill dependency. For insomniacs, life is a constant struggle because of the accumulative effects of long-term sleep deprivation.

Health issues abound, depression becomes a major risk, their ability to function normally is often impaired, and they lose sight of their potential to deal successfully with life's daily challenges. They sometimes refer to their condition as living in a nightmare world where they are constantly exhausted and simply cannot function. It's completely understandable that a doctor would prescribe sleeping drugs because the dangers of sleep deprivation can be acute.

Before we begin to examine the practicalities of sleep, we need to know how much sleep is appropriate for each of us as individuals. It's not surprising that different age groups have different sleep requirements.

For example, very young children and infants can sleep in total for around 14 - 15 hours a day. And if you've got teenagers, you might have guessed that adolescents usually need more sleep than adults. Teens can easily sleep between 8.5 to 9.5 hours a night.

It's widely understood that during the first trimester, pregnant women often find they need a lot more sleep than usual. The fact is that if you feel tired during the day, find yourself yawning or taking a nap, you're short on sleep. And this is the time for you to do something practical, realistic, and effective to take care of the problem.

There are many myths surrounding the condition known as OAS or Obstructive Sleep Apnea. It's estimated that around 18 million Americans suffer from the condition but the numbers could be much higher because many people don't report the condition to their doctors. This condition is far more than just loud snoring, although snoring can be a sign of sleep apnea.

People with this condition skip breathing 400 times during the night. The delay in breathing can last from ten to thirty seconds and is then followed by a loud snore as breathing suddenly resumes. The normal sleep cycle is interrupted and this can leave sufferers feeling tired and exhausted during the day. It is a serious condition, especially since it can lead to accidents at work, problems when driving, as well as increasing the risk of heart attacks and strokes. It can affect people of all ages, including children, but tends to affect people more after the age of forty.

Weight also plays a part and there is evidence that shedding excess pounds can improve the condition. Despite all the advice and overwhelming evidence, there are still surprising numbers of sleep apnea sufferers who continue to smoke. Smoking is a perfect way to increase the severity and risks of this debilitating condition.

If you've already trimmed your weight, quit smoking and tried sleeping on your side but still suffer from the condition, you need to see your doctor. There are many treatments available including a special mask that delivers constant air flow to keep the breathing passage open. Lifestyle choices can clearly make a positive difference, too.

Your body, your brain, your mind and your emotional functioning all rely on sufficient sleep to operate efficiently. If you don't get enough sleep, everything suffers. Research suggests that it's much harder than you might imagine to adapt having less sleep than your body needs. The sleep deficit has to be repaid at some point or we'll experience increasingly severe problems.

Simple techniques of preparing for bed

1. Try to get to bed early. The recharging of the body's adrenal system usually takes place between 11p.m. and 1a.m. in the morning. The gallbladder uses the same time to release the toxin build up in the body. If you happen to be awake when both these functions are taking place within your body, there is the possibility of the toxin backing up to the liver which can endanger your health very badly. Sleeping late are byproducts of

modern living styles. However, the human body was created in synchronization of nature and its activities. That is why before the advent of electricity people used to go to bed just after sundown and wake up with sunrise.

2. Don't alter your bedtimes haphazardly. Try to stick to a pattern where you go to bed and wake up at the same time. This should be done even on weekends. The continuous pattern will help your body to fit into a rhythm.

3. Maintain a soothing bedtime routine. This can change from person to person. You can use deep breathing exercises, meditation, use of aromatherapy, a gentle relaxing massage given by your partner, or even going through a complete and relaxing skin care routine. The secret is to get into a rhythm which makes you comfortable, relaxed, and ready for bed. Repeating it every day will help in easing out the tensions of the day.

4. Refrain from taking any heavy fluids two hours before bed time. This habit will minimize the number of times you need to visit the bathroom in the middle of the night. You should also make a habit of going to the bathroom just before you get into bed, so that you will not get the urge during night time.

5. Eat a meal enriched with proteins several hours before your bed time. The protein will enhance the production of L-tryptophan which is essential for the production of serotonin and melatonin. Follow up your meal with some fruit to help the tryptophan to cross easily across the blood brain barrier.

6. Refrain from taking any snacks while in bed or just before bed and reduce the level of sugar and grains in your dinner time as it

will raise the blood sugar level, delaying sleep. When the body starts metabolizing these elements and the blood sugar level start dropping you will find yourself suddenly awake and unable to go back to sleep.

7. A hot bath before bed is found to be very soothing. When the body temperature is stimulated to a raised level during late evening by the time you get into bed, it will be ready to drop, signaling slumber time to your brain.

8. Stop your work and put them away ideally one to two hours before bed. The interval between work and bedtime should be used for unwinding from the pressure and tension of work. It is essential that you approach your bed with a calm mind instead of being hyped up about some matter.

9. If you prefer reading, a novel with an uplifting story instead of a stimulating one like suspense or mystery is recommended. Or the suspense will keep you up half the night awake trying to visualize the end to the mystery!

A Few Lifestyle Suggestions to Make You Sleep Better

Don't take medications and drugs unless it is absolutely necessary for your health and wellbeing. A majority of prescribed and over the counter drugs can cause changes in your sleeping patterns.

Avoid drinks with alcohol or caffeine. Caffeine takes longer to metabolize in the body so that your body will experience its effects much longer after consumption. That is why even the cup of coffee you had in the evening will keep you awake during the night. Some of the medications and drugs in the market also contain caffeine which account for their capacity to generate sleeping irregularities. Though alcohol can make you feel drowsy the effect is very much short lived. Once the feeling goes away, you will find that sleep is eluding you for many hours and even the sleep that you finally reach will not take you to deep slumber after alcohol. In the absence of deep sleep, your body will not be able to perform its usual healing and regeneration process is vital for lasting healthiness.

Engage in regular exercise activities. If you are contained in an 8-hour office job, you should make sure that your body receives plenty of exercise which can dramatically increase your sleep health. The best time to exercise is, however, not closer to your bedtime but in the morning.

Keep away from sensitive food types that will keep you awake at night like sugar, pasteurized dairy foods, and grains. These foods can result in congestion, leading to gastric disorders.

The sleep apnea risk is enhanced amongst people with weight issues. If you think you have gained a few extra pounds and during this time you have also experienced sleeping trouble focus on losing the extra weight as a priority. The sleeping issue will correct automatically.

If your body is going through a hormone upheaval like during menopausal or premenopausal time, seek advice from your family physician, as this time can lead to sleeping difficulties.

Want to read more? Purchase our book on **Effective Guide On How to Sleep Well Everyday** *today!*

References

ALPHA BOOKS. (2019). *HEAL YOURSELF WITH CBD OIL*. [Place of publication not identified]: ALPHA Books.

Dube, E. (n.d.). *CBD oil and hemp oil.*

Harris, J. (n.d.). *Hemp oil & CBD.*

Lidicker, G. (n.d.). *CBD oil: everyday secrets.*

Mindell, E. (n.d.). *Healing with hemp CBD oil.*

Nelson, X. (n.d.). *CBD Hemp Oil.*

Rappaport, T. and Leonard-Johnson, S. (n.d.). *CBD-rich hemp oil.*

Rosenthal, T. (n.d.). *CBD hemp oil 101.*

Stevens, R. (n.d.). *CBD oil for pain relief.*

www.ingramcontent.com/pod-product-compliance
Lightning Source LLC
Chambersburg PA
CBHW051351280526
45784CB00007B/2914